The
Intimacy
Solution

Life Lessons in Sex and Love

Erika Schwartz, MD

Post Hill
PRESS

A POST HILL PRESS BOOK
ISBN: 978-1-68261-746-5
ISBN (eBook): 978-1-68261-747-2

The Intimacy Solution:
Life Lessons in Sex and Love

This book contains advice and information relating to health care. It
should be used to supplement rather than replace the advice of your
doctor or another trained health professional. If you know or suspect
that you have a health problem, it is recommended that you seek
your physician's advice before embarking on any medical program or
treatment. All efforts have been made to assure the accuracy of the
information in this book as of the date of publication. The publisher
and the author disclaim liability for any medical outcomes that may
occur as a result of applying the methods suggested in this book.

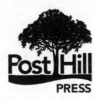

Post Hill Press
New York • Nashville
posthillpress.com

Published in the United States of America

*To my patients and friends, thank you for
generously sharing your love stories with me.
They will give many clearer insights into matters
of sex and intimacy.*

(All names have been changed to protect the not so innocent.)

ACKNOWLEDGMENTS

The Intimacy Solution is a compilation of intimate stories told to me by patients and friends and the insights and life lessons gained from them. I want to thank all for being so honest and generous, for sharing your intimate secrets with me, and giving me a bird's eye view into your individual sexuality and its connection to love.

Thank you, Anthony Ziccardi, for being the most supportive, fun publisher and good friend.

Thank you, Gene, for all the invaluable help and your devoted love for my four-legged muses.

Thank you, Lisa and Katie, for teaching me how crucial it is to openly share even TMI between generations so we can learn from one another how to navigate the turbulent waters of personal relationships.

Thank you, Matt and Gordon, for your priceless input on the youngish male perspectives on marriage and relationships.

To Wendy, Rhonda, and Linda, thank you for your insights into staying forever young, passionate, and sexy.

Thank you, Michael Nitti, for helping both men and women become the best versions of themselves in life and relationships. Your optimism and compassion make the world a better place. Keep teaching us.

To Jack, Taylor, Paige, Lucy, and Nellie, I hope by the time you get to puberty and adolescence the lessons of this book are common knowledge and intimacy is no longer such a mystery.

CONTENTS

CHAPTER 1

WHAT'S SEX
GOT TO DO WITH IT?

"I don't know the question,
but sex is definitely the answer."

—Woody Allen

Television shows. The internet. Social media. Hollywood's biggest movies. Magazine covers. Billboards. Commercials. Department store windows. All around us, every aspect of our culture reminds us that sex is at the very heart of what it means to be human. Just like eating, sleeping, and breathing, sex is an omnipresent part of our everyday lives.

What these constant cues fail to reveal, however, is what sex is supposed to *mean* to us as individuals as we struggle to make sense of an increasingly complex modern world.

There's a reason for this—it's because sex doesn't have one simple definition. Throughout life's twists and turns, sex means different things, ranging from pure animal attraction and lust to the deepest levels of intimacy and love. It can represent the heart of a loving relationship or an expression of anger; a symbol of power, a weapon, or the closest two people can ever get to reaching total understanding and empathy with each other.

As a physician specializing in internal medicine, trauma, bioidentical hormone treatments, age management, and disease prevention, I have come to understand how sex spans the entire spectrum of human emotion and life stages, how it connects to intimacy, and how it affects everything we do in our lives, as I'll illustrate throughout this book with many personal stories from patients and friends. Depending on infinite variables—including age, gender, situational and environmental factors—the way we express our sexuality either helps to expand and give our lives more depth or disappoints and frustrates us, draining our precious energy, leaving us bereft and empty without closeness or intimacy.

In more than 35 years of caring for people, I have had the great privilege to follow thousands of patients of all ages through their lives and sexual journeys, and listen to their most intimate stories of how sex and sexuality have touched and shaped their lives and even careers. No two people are alike, and no two stories are the same. While every tale is unique, I have observed a common thread winding through them all, regardless of cultural mores, life situations, or personal expectations. This common thread unites us all in our individual interpretations of intimacy and offers ways to better understand ourselves, how sex drives us, and how intimacy and sex are connected (or not) at different ages and stages of our lives. I've divided these stages of sex and intimacy into the four "seasons" of sexuality: **spring**, **summer**, **fall**, and **winter**.

THE FOUR SEASONS OF SEX

As every middle school health teacher will tell you, teenagers are driven by hormones. This time is our sexual **spring**. During adolescence, our sex hormones—estrogen, progesterone, testosterone, and of course pheromones—start flowing through our bodies. Not only do we transition from little kids to men and women physically but on a psychological and emotional level we morph into sexual human beings. There are some exceptions to the rule, of course, but in general, the blind desire to seek out and have sex is the prime motivator during the teenage sexual spring years.

It feels like endless **summer** as we enter adulthood. In our 20s and 30s, the same hormones that made us sex-crazy as teens now drive us to reproduce. In evolutionary terms, it's all about the genetic imperative, survival of our species. In this instance as well, all roads also lead to sex. Whether we identify our sexual orientation as straight, gay, lesbian, pansexual, queer, bi, or other, the culture generally equates our sex drive during these years with the search for love and intimacy. This is the period when we seek relationships that have meaning to us, because as humans we need love and intimacy to couple up, mate, and form families in the quest to fulfill our physiologic mandate— the perpetuation of our species.

Once children enter the picture, however, sex enters the back-to-school atmosphere of **fall**, as relationships between couples become more complex and more unpredictable. Sexuality led by hormones alone is no longer front and center. Things aren't that simple anymore. Men and women in modern marriages or partnerships shift their focus due to continuously changing pressures and demands associated with raising and supporting a family, and the hot sex that brought them together in the first place invariably takes a back seat. In the hustle and bustle of family life, couples often forget or don't even realize that when sex goes missing from a marriage, intimacy and connection often go with it. Our culture offers no tools to help relationships without sex last, and regardless of how impossible it becomes to accomplish, sex is still considered the defining factor of success in relationships and the determinant of intimacy. Sociological pressures to maintain the family unit and the memories of the passion that brought couples together often help them to hang in there during this potentially disruptive time. Kids may help keep couples together during this phase, as do deeper aspects of love, commitment, and friendship, along with the still very-much-present hormones, but also simply comfort, force of habit and the cultural morays contribute.

Once the kids are grown, the free time and privacy necessary to bring sex back into a relationship may bring passion back, but by then hormones are no longer the driving force. As both men and women enter the next phase in life—menopause for women and andropause for men—production of sex hormones wanes, making sex an item of lesser importance on the daily to-do list.

Even when the desire strikes, many men and women find themselves far less physically and emotionally aroused, less able or willing to perform the way they did in their youth. Now in the **winter** of sexuality, everyone gets hit face-on with the reality of this unexpected yet highly significant sea change in the relationship. Either the two have grown together, maintained, or even increased their togetherness, intimacy, friendship, and trust and are able to find ways to rekindle the sexual fire, as well as redefine the role of sex and how it can serve to keep their relationship alive—or there isn't much of a relationship left. At this point, oftentimes one or both of the partners may have already moved on, emotionally or physically or both. This is the make-or-break point, when many find that a relationship expected to last a lifetime was built on a foundation of sand. Many find that it's better just to walk away and take the lesson learned than live a lie that will only make for more loneliness and misery in old age.

In subsequent chapters, we'll delve more deeply into each of these complex and mysterious seasons and mysteries of sex and their connection to intimacy and love. I hope the wide variety of stories I will share with you, people I've laughed and cried with, and always cheered on over the years—from teens to people in their 70s and beyond—will serve to help you better understand your own sexuality and gain better insight into what you want your future to be and how to make it your ideal reality. In each chapter, you'll find lessons and tools my patients and I have found useful to improve not only sexuality but also emotional awareness, to help reach the gold ring of where sex and love meet in your personal journey.

CULTURE VERSUS HORMONES

It may be hormones that drive the physiology of our sexual behavior, but culture determines how we express it. William Masters and Virginia Johnson were among the first to attempt to quantify scientifically what happens physiologically during the act of sex. Their work broke ground, opened some minds and shattered old stereotypes that kept people in the dark about sexuality for centuries. But their research, albeit invaluable, is clinical and scientifically disconnected from reality. Unfortunately, it's also terribly out of date. Their information tried to separate sex from emotion and as a result failed in the important defining details of our sexuality: the connection to intimacy, love, and emotional closeness. It's amazing to me that even today, six decades later, confusion, fear, and misinformation too often still rule our sex lives and decisions we make surrounding sex. The *Masters of Sex* TV show, which focuses on the story of Masters and Johnson and their work, is a reminder of how our medical profession has looked at and still does look at sexuality, purely as a physiologic act. It helps therapists remember the science and the history of sex, but it doesn't help you and me have better sex or get emotionally any closer to our partners. It certainly does not help any of us learn what intimacy means nor how to connect it to sex.

Before Masters and Johnson, Alfred Kinsey published his findings on male sexuality in the late 1940s. He also failed to make the emotional connection, thus leaving us with little insight into the connection between sex and emotion.

Consider some of these still common and often harmful misconceptions hovering around both men and women despite all the research into sexuality:

- Unless you are constantly interested in sex and thinking about it all the time, you're not normal.
- If your sex life doesn't mimic what you see on reality TV, media, celebrity lives, and in the movies, you're doing something wrong or you're just a misfit.
- Unless sex is about love and intimacy regardless of age and time of life, it is just porn.
- Children and teens learn about sex mostly from their friends and the media. They're not really affected by the examples they see at home.
- It's okay for women to be sexually active and promiscuous while they're young, because it helps them be popular and proves they're equal to men.
- Everyone is having mind-blowing sex all the time, and if you're not, you'll never fit in and never be really happy—not to mention, you aren't normal.
- Everyone must get married and have kids in order to have a complete and satisfying life.
- Monogamy means one partner for life, and if you don't follow this dogma, you've failed and there is something wrong with you.
- Only the young have passionate sex lives. Once you're old, you might as well take up gardening or knitting.

Sex is only for the young and beautiful with perfect bodies.

- Only women go through menopause and then don't care about sex anymore, while men want and can have sex at any age, explaining why older men leave their older wives for younger women.
- Only men go through midlife crises.

These blanket statements cause people to worry about what other people think and follow other people's paths no matter how unhappy it may make them. When we accept cultural and social stereotypes as our destinies, we end up in marriages that may look picture-perfect from the outside but feel desperately empty underneath; we fake smiles for the camera, we fake orgasms for our partners, and we fake happiness for ourselves. We sleepwalk through the only life we've got. I've met people who lived for decades in shame and secrecy until they learned that sexuality is as individual as each one of us. The information I've gathered over decades of clinical practice must be shared, because it provides a refreshingly different, sometimes raw but realistic and honest perspective on sexuality at all ages and under a variety of circumstances. The information and stories I'll share with you have helped my patients and me lead more accepting, tolerant, kind, and happy lives, and I hope they will help you too.

To make things clearer, I've broken sexuality down into three most important components:

§ **Hormones.** As we go into puberty, our sex hormones—estrogen, progesterone, and testosterone—wake up, and when that alarm clock goes off, we suddenly become sexual beings. Pheromones fly, sex occupies practically every minute of our thoughts, and having sex becomes our raison d'etre. Later, as adults, we also experience hormone changes that significantly affect our sexuality. The impact of our hormones and their effects is a recurring theme in this book.

§ **Environment/culture.** Our first sexual role models are our parents. How they interact and how their sexuality intertwines with the degree of intimacy between them define how we view sex and intimacy as young children and later on as adults. Along with what we see at home is what we see in the world around us. We are all deeply affected by the internet, social media, movies, TV, and print media. All these elements contribute to various degrees to the formation of our sexual identities, the connections to intimacy, and the role sex plays in our everyday lives.

§ **Personal truth.** Despite how our culture indoctrinates us, we are all individuals, with different needs, desires, turn-ons and turnoffs—likes and dislikes. I describe personal truth as a combination of genetic makeup, body-mind self-perception, sexuality, and unique perspective. The environmental and physiologic factors noted above play significant roles. These influences make their presence felt at every phase of our sexual lives but we are all individuals and must find our own individual truth about sex and intimacy. I'll show you how outside influences derail us and give you insights to help you identify the root causes of confusion and the tools to create clarity. My goal is to help you find your personal truth and make your life better and easier.

ALL PEOPLE SEEM TO HAVE GREAT SEX ALL THE TIME. AM I THE ONLY ONE WHO ISN'T?

I'll answer that in three words: They are *not*. Feel better?

We all dream about having more of that unique form of temporary insanity and abandon that passionate sex brings into our lives, and it's the job of the media and entertainment factories to serve us our fantasies on a silver platter on an ongoing basis everywhere we turn. But what we see in the movies, on the internet, and on TV; what we read about in erotic novels or in the advice columns of *Cosmopolitan* and *Esquire*—even the bragging we hear from our close friends—is usually just fantasy.

Let's take a 2014 article in the newspaper *The Guardian* reporting on the National Survey of Sexual Attitudes and Lifestyles in England for instance. Of 15,000 British adults who responded, 19.5 percent of men and 20 percent of women ages 25 to 34 hadn't had sex in the previous month, and 21.1 percent of men and 27.9 percent of women ages 45 to 54 reported a minimum of a four-week sexual dry spell. On average, women reported an 8 percent higher abstinence rate than men.[1] In a

Woman's Day survey, only 48 percent of Americans reported being satisfied with their sex lives.[2]

So take a deep breath out and relax. Your sex life is your sex life, and you don't need to compare it to the action the women on *Sex and the City* or the vampires on *True Blood* are getting, or at least are saying they are. Isn't that a comforting thing to know? It's nice to know life is more like *House of Cards* (well, maybe not the threesome) and *Breaking Bad* or *Ozark* than those hot and steamy sex scenes on *Scandal*.

THERE IS MUCH MORE TO SEX THAN THE BODY

While our sex hormones are crucial ingredients in the making of our sex drives and interests, our mating patterns, parental examples, and friends, along with socialization and society's expectations, mold the shape of our adult sexuality. But it is ultimately the individual relationship, the two people having sex, that determines whether or not a particular sexual bond will turn into the kind of intimacy that will last through the realities of a lifetime.

Many of our perceived or real sexual problems are created by our culture, society, sociology and of course, friends and family. Low or no libido may mask homosexual, asexual, transsexual, or polysexual drives that in some cultures or groups are still considered unacceptable. People who are afraid to come out of the closet, sometimes for good reasons (societal pressures, bullying, and threats) often choose to deny their entire sexuality by suppressing their sexual impulses. This can make them appear strange or different, since an active and high sex drive is the cultural expectation for youth. Compounded with the self-perception of being a misfit if unable to lead a highly sexual life often leads to depression, drug and alcohol abuse, multiple unexplained medical problems, and even suicide.

While understanding how a group of individuals thinks and how their thought processes determine behavior is very important, I've noticed over decades of practice that most of us feel and behave differently than the group. Every situation, with its specific quirks and twists, is unique. To a kind and caring physician who asks the right questions, every patient will happily open up and share a miraculous personal world that may help the doctor aid the patient better navigate life's stormy waters.

One question—implicitly asked in the title of this chapter—is, what's all the fuss about sex, after all? Sex is supposed to be the be-all and end-all, the sun around which the planets of our lives and relationships rotate. Most of my patients believe this to be a fact, and this is why they become so distressed and ashamed when they feel they aren't living up to our society's astronomical sexual expectations.

So, what's sex got to do with it? I have a patient who has answered that question in a very unexpected way. Take a moment and consider her story.

Lucy first came to me as a patient when she was 28. At the time, I was practicing internal medicine in a suburb of New York City, a town she lived in. She was an attractive, slim, healthy young woman whom I saw for annual physicals. She was a long-distance runner, so, once in a while, she'd come in with strained muscles or a sprained ankle; maybe a cold or virus occasionally.

Over the years, we became friends, going out together socially and meeting each other's families. One day Lucy told me that when she was in her early 20s, her college boyfriend broke her heart. They'd never had sex, but they were close emotionally for over three years, and, in her perception, they were dating exclusively and seriously. She still seemed sad when she talked about him a decade later. Lucy came from a religious family and told me she had always believed in waiting until marriage to have sex. To her, sex and intimacy were one, so she had waited to marry this man she had loved in her youth. Since that relationship didn't work out, she just stayed single. Her life was full and she was a happy and a well-adjusted woman.

Gradually, over the course of a few years, I noticed that whenever we got together with a group of female friends to share the usual stories of dating, engagements, and marriages, Lucy never seemed interested in sharing any story involving sex. Over the years, she never dated anyone and refused to allow any of her friends to fix her up. In time, as the rest of us paired off, Lucy stayed single. At weddings and special occasions, she sometimes brought along different guys, whom she always introduced as a friend from work or the gym. Over the decades I knew Lucy, she never dated either men or women.

As time went by, Lucy always appeared content and didn't show any sign of depression, and never verbalized any concern over the lack of a man in her life.

Do I feel sorry for Lucy? Absolutely not! In fact, she is probably one of the most cheerful, vital people I know. She has a highly successful and stressful job, at which she excels. She owns her own home where she lives with her two beloved dogs, and she has a close circle of male and female friends. Lucy never wanted nor talked about having children either, but she is a loving and involved aunt and a godmother to two of her friends' children. When she went into menopause, she came to me for hormones to help her feel better and potentially forestall diseases of ageing. Never once in the decades of knowing her have I heard her complain or appear unhappy or unfulfilled.

I share Lucy's story because she defies so many stereotypes. By her own choice, she is living a satisfying, fulfilling life—without sex. Lucy is an example of many people I have seen who don't seem to be moved by the hormone storm of teen years, nor by the need to mate and create a family with children to leave as legacy. I call people like Lucy asexual. Some people call her part of "the fourth sexual orientation,"[3] and we're starting to see strong evidence in the medical and scientific literature of happily sexless people. These men and women are not pansexual, since they don't demonstrate interest or sexually charged affection toward any particular gender. In fact, maybe it's as simple as the fact that their emotional growth may have stopped before puberty, and I personally believe that is why hormones do not affect them or change their outlook on life or bring sexuality to their front burner.

I've had arguments with colleagues who claim asexuals don't exist at all—that they're mythical creatures, like unicorns. They believe asexuals are suppressed or repressed gay, lesbian, or transgender people. I disagree, and, fortunately, so do many cutting-edge researchers. In our society, where sexuality is no longer solely a gender issue and where acceptance of individual preference is finally becoming the norm, I believe it is time to accept people who have never developed a taste or need for sexual expression. They are normal. They function well, and they don't feel the need to fit into our society by defining themselves through their sexuality. To people who are not interested in sex, intimacy may easily be found in their relationships with friends, family, and pets. Maybe there is nothing wrong with being able to separate sex from intimacy when the separation doesn't hurt anyone.

Why begin a book about sex and intimacy with a story of a person who doesn't have interest in sex yet experiences intimacy in other aspects of her life? Because it is a perfect example of what I identify as a personal truth. Each of us is unique. We're all as different in our preferences for sex and intimacy as snowflakes in a storm. Lucy's story illustrates what I'll stress again and again throughout this book: Sexuality at any stage of life isn't a paint-by-numbers project. The key to a healthy and emotionally fulfilling sex life comes directly from our ability to listen to our bodies and hearts, and then to be honest with ourselves.

THE SEXUALITY PUZZLE

Sexuality is extremely complex, and in this book, I've tried to put together some pieces of this puzzle. Age, genetics, health, cultural and sociological factors, the media, peers, group behavior, and many other influences are all ingredients in this fascinating mystery. As you read on, you'll discover that:

- Sexuality is one of the most complicated—and least understood—parts of our lives. It's also among the most difficult to research.
- There is a direct and indelible interaction between hormones and sexual and emotional behavior.
- Sexual problems at any age are not unusual, and they are also not necessarily insurmountable.
- Although you are unique as a person, you are not alone with the problems you face. Never be ashamed or embarrassed. There is always someone with a similar story who can identify with you, share with you, and validate you.
- Viewing sex in the context of health and culture and then applying it to your personal situation is crucial to finding balance and a satisfying life.
- Sexuality continues but changes dramatically throughout life.
- Sexual identity and tendencies may fluctuate throughout life.
- If you don't feel the need to make sex the centerpiece of your life, it doesn't mean something's wrong with you.
- Being able to connect sexuality to intimacy at various stages of life will lead you to a more satisfying and emotionally healthier life than separating sex from intimacy.

Today, we are living longer than ever before, and as the beaming gray-haired couples in the Viagra ads constantly remind us, we're expected to keep enjoying sex well into our golden years. In order to live up to this image of eternal sexual vigor if we so choose, it behooves us to examine more closely the roles that sexuality, intimacy, and relationships play in our lives. The better we understand ourselves, the better we will communicate in love and sex, and the more likely it is we can live fulfilling lives with truly intimate relationships.

Before you dive further into this book, keep this in mind: While we all have much in common biologically and culturally, we are individuals, and we experience life and sex in unique ways. Our reactions and perspectives are our own, and no two of us are alike. There's a saying in 12-step groups regarding the personal testimonials that are the centerpiece of their meetings: "Identify but don't compare." Please consider this as you read the personal stories, and use the information in the book to help you learn and put your own sexuality and intimacy into perspective. I sincerely hope this book will help you better understand your own sexuality, at whatever age or stage of life you are.

CHAPTER 2

YOUR SEXUAL SELF: HOW IT DEVELOPS

"Sex is emotion in motion."

—Mae West

Here I am, in the second chapter of a book about sex, and we haven't even sorted out a proper definition of "sexuality." That's because it's not as simple as it seems. Everyone is trying to tell us something different about what sexuality is. Psychiatrists try to address the emotional aspects of sexuality, while sociologists study its cultural implications. Anthropologists pour over the historical data, while sexologists investigate the act. Add in the misinformation and many lies about sex fed to us by the media, internet, family, and friends—not to mention the lies we tell ourselves—and you've got a situation ripe for conflict and confusion.

I think perhaps Mae West—the curvaceous siren of the early silver screen—said it best in the quote beginning this chapter: "Sex is emotion in motion." Even though her heyday was in the

1920s, Mae could teach us a thing or two about sex today. She understood that sex isn't any one thing. It's far more than simply a physical act or process. Sure, your body—how it looks and functions—is a major player. Your hormones and your age are supporting actors too. But these are just at the top of a long list of contributing factors that impact—and even determine—how you will express your sexuality and how satisfied and content you will be throughout the different seasons of your life. The meaning of sex changes over the course of our lives and the better we understand ourselves, the more we will be able to interpret the significance of the changes and adjust accordingly.

Since sex drive starts with an awakening of sex hormones, an explanation of the role the endocrine system plays in sexuality is a good place to start our quest for a deeper understanding of sexuality.

THE HORMONE CONNECTION

Hormones directly affect all our bodily functions and actions. Yet the role of hormones is confusing and sadly underestimated, for many reasons. The most significant one is that we cannot see them. To the general public—and sadly, to plenty of my colleagues in the medical profession—the function and interaction of hormones in the body seem vague and difficult to grasp. We just don't get much training about hormones outside disease states.

There are at least three broad categories of hormones that play significant roles in our bodies and our lives. The first is naturally occurring hormones: substances produced by the body itself. The second includes hormones that come from the air we breathe, the food we eat, the medications we take, as well as those that get into our cells through other external means. The third is substances the medical profession calls "hormones" that are chemicals made to have hormone-like effects and trick our bodies into believing they are hormones. (Reference my book *The New Hormone Solution* for more details.) These are what people who understand hormones call "hormone impostors." They include birth control pills, certain forms of nonbioidentical hormone replacement therapy (HRT), and anabolic steroids used by bodybuilders and even some professional athletes. The problem is that many doctors and laypeople don't know the distinction between real hormones and hormone impostors. They believe all hormone preparations have the same effects, and this is incorrect and causes problems. Regardless of age, we all need balanced hormones to stay healthy and to look and feel great.

NATURAL HORMONES—THE HORMONES YOUR BODY MAKES

Human sexuality is directly defined by three primary sex hormones: estrogen, progesterone, and testosterone. These hormones are present in both men and women in different quantities, at different stages of life. As I shared in my book *The New Hormone Solution*, every cell in our bodies has receptors for hormones, and if the proper hormone attaches to the correct receptor, the result is a balanced, healthy person. While I will try to explain the roles of these hormones separately, please understand they all work together—their effects interact and affect the outcome together, not individually.

Estrogen is the main female sex hormone. It defines females as they go from childhood, where there is no identifiable physiological difference between males and females, to puberty. At puberty, there is suddenly increased production of estrogen by the ovaries, adrenal glands (small glands situated on top of the kidneys) and fat cells. As a result, breast buds develop, perspiration has adult odor, and pubic and armpit hair starts to grow culminating with the start of menstruation. Estrogen defines the physical transition from girl to woman.

As girls become adults, estrogen makes things grow on the inside of the body as well. Breasts develop and the lining of the uterus thickens in preparation for implantation of a fertilized egg when pregnancy occurs. Estrogen also affects the brain by stimulating serotonin production, leading to good mood and optimistic outlook and helps women identify themselves as women. The highest concentration of estrogen receptors in the female body are found in the heart, brain, bones, and sexual organs. That's why when a woman has a hysterectomy (removal of the uterus) and her ovaries are removed as well, it is imperative that she receives estrogen supplementation to keep her heart, brain, and other organs from falling apart.

Estrogen works closely with **progesterone**. This hormone is produced by a temporary organ called the corpus luteum, which develops after ovulation when an egg is pushed out into the Fallopian tubes on its way to the uterus. The corpus luteum, left behind in the ovary where the egg has been extruded (tossed out), produces progesterone. This is the hormone that balances the effects of estrogen (good and bad). One of its many roles is to prepare the lining of the uterus, the endometrium, for implantation of a fertilized egg and to help keep the egg safely implanted in the uterine lining so it can develop into a fetus. Progesterone also affects the balance of water in the body and hormone production in the brain. It helps keeps the brain calm and minimizes symptoms of PMS. Progesterone affects sugar metabolism and all the other hormones. When progesterone is low or out of balance with estrogen, most women feel off-kilter, don't sleep well, and often become irritable and anxious.

Testosterone is the most abundant sex hormone in women throughout their lives. Men and women differ in the quantity of testosterone they produce; women manufacture much lower quantities than men. In women, testosterone is produced in the ovaries and adrenals. All hormones in women are produced in pulses, released from the pituitary gland in the brain down to the sex hormones. No human in the physiologic state lives with constant or continuous hormone levels.

Although the ovarian cycle was first described in the 1930s, we still don't know everything about our sex hormones—but we do know that the role of testosterone in women is critical. While it's often difficult to distinguish between some of the effects of how important testosterone is. There's more information about testosterone to be found in pop literature than in medical education. In my 35-plus years of experience with more than 50,000 patients, I sometimes see middle-aged women in new relationships who—despite low testosterone levels in their blood—have a strong libido and do not experience vaginal dryness. The driver in these women is the excitement of the new relationship, not the testosterone level. A low testosterone level may cause anxiety, depression, and fatigue. Scientific data on women and men demonstrates that testosterone not only balances estrogen but it may also help prevent breast cancer, heart disease, and even Alzheimer's. Sadly, the medical profession doesn't know loss of muscle mass as well as loss of libido may be directly connected to loss of testosterone.

In contrast, in practices like mine, in which the focus is to help men and women feel great and prevent disease, testosterone supplementation is pretty standard. Testosterone increases muscle mass (strong muscles protect the bones and help prevent osteoporosis) something no drug can effectively or safely do. Testosterone boosts mood and confidence in both genders too. But be warned: The kind of testosterone therapy prescribed for women is a lower dose than the dose needed for men. (Women, please don't use your man's supply of testosterone, unless you want to grow facial hair, get acne around your jawline, develop a baritone voice, develop clitoral enlargement, or find yourself with a sex drive that may be out of control.) Since testosterone is not available in FDA-approved formulations for women and must be compounded to provide appropriate doses and preparations for women, always work with a doctor who knows how to prescribe hormones in wellness and disease prevention, and who has extensive experience with compounding, to get optimum benefits and no undesirable side effects.

Men make the same hormones. They need estrogen to feel good, prevent heart disease, build muscle, maintain a positive outlook on life, and of course, maintain their libido. However, the difference between men and women is in the amounts of hormones they produce. Men at their physiologic peak make somewhere between 100 to 500 times more testosterone than women if they are healthy and sexual, build muscle, maintain a generally good mood, keep weight off, and get erections that are strong enough and last long enough to provide them with satisfactory sex lives and the ability to have intercourse. The adrenal glands and testicles make progesterone in men as well. While the amounts are very low compared to women, the impact of progesterone is important in providing balance for the metabolites (byproducts of breakdown) of testosterone, which may be toxic. These undesirable metabolic byproducts include DHT (dihydrotestosterone), known to cause hair loss, weight gain, and increased inflammation in men as they age, making them susceptible to heart disease and other diseases of aging, such as Alzheimer's, diabetes, and arthritis.

Hormones aren't just for sexual function. Every minute of every day, there is a fully orchestrated symphony being performed inside our bodies, involving thousands of different hormones. For instance, insulin affects blood sugar levels. When you eat a meal and the food is digested and then absorbed into the bloodstream, the products of digestion include sugars (carbohydrates, or carbs) that turn into glucose in the bloodstream and stimulate the production of insulin by the pancreas. The role of insulin is to drive the sugar into the cells of organs, providing them with nourishment allowing them to function optimally. Extra glucose is stored in the liver. But insulin—like all the other hormones—doesn't perform alone. Its partners are estrogen, progesterone, testosterone, cortisol, serotonin, dopamine, aldosterone, renin, thyroid and many other hormones. With age, poor diet, environmental toxins, and sedentary lifestyles, people often develop what is known as insulin resistance, the precursor not only of diabetes but also of cancer and other chronic diseases of aging.

Hormones also control blood pressure, arterial resistance, and flexibility. Renin and angiotensin are two hormones produced in the kidneys and lungs. They determine how our arteries react to the blood flowing through them. Along with the adrenal hormone aldosterone arteries contract in response to these hormones and cause high blood pressure, renal failure, and other significant disease states. Dietary changes, medication and exercise can help improve the hormone balance helping prevent strokes and heart attacks. And, like the other hormones, renin, aldosterone, and angiotensin don't ever work alone. Estrogen, progesterone, and testosterone, as well as cortisol and insulin, are integral parts of this ever-expanding orchestra.

Cortisol is the "fight or flight" hormone. Made in the adrenal glands it is released every time the brain perceives danger. Its release causes blood flow to be redirected to muscles and bones, to make us run faster; increases heart rate and releases adrenalin; stops us from thinking about sex; and shifts our focus to survival. Again, estrogen, progesterone, and testosterone, along with insulin, serotonin, dopamine, and many others affect cortisol production and work together to protect us from real or perceived danger.

Serotonin and dopamine, the most studied of the feel-good hormones—called neurotransmitters—produced by the brain, are important for our survival and our ability to enjoy life without constantly feeling depressed, under a cloud, and paralyzed by overwhelming anxiety and the inability to accomplish day-to-day tasks. Their interaction with estrogen, progesterone, and testosterone is crucial to our mood and sexual balance. High serotonin and dopamine levels make us feel great, while low levels leave us depressed, uninterested in sex, and just plain unhappy. When estrogen and testosterone are at optimum levels, we rarely get depressed unless there is a real tragedy affecting our lives. So when you think of mood disorders and how to treat them, remember the root cause is low levels of serotonin, dopamine, and other neurotransmitter hormones, not a deficiency of antidepressants. Most patients I see on antidepressants have diminished sex drives and too often lead medicated and emotionally disconnected lives.

Hormones are the crucial factors in maintaining optimum health for all men and women, so why do they get such a bad rap? Women blame those poor invisible hormones for everything from headaches to hot flashes to loss of libido. Men love to call an emotional woman "hormonal." Part of my mission as a hormone doctor and author is to shatter stereotypes and correct as much misinformation as possible. Hormones play such a positive role in our lives that their importance cannot be overstated. They keep us healthy and feeling well. When estrogen, progesterone, testosterone, and all the other hormones are in balance, we glow. Our weight is optimal and easy to maintain, we think clearly, and our outlook on life in general is optimistic. We are sexually charged and raring to go, releasing pheromones that make us sexually attractive. Our skin is soft, our reproductive systems are humming, and the world is full of possibilities. When our hormones are in balance, we feel alive—we are young. And how often are young people victims of cancer and heart attacks? Not as often as the aged.

It is the *lack* or *imbalance* of hormones that causes us to feel old, gain weight, lose libido and lapse into sedentary and elderly behavior. Without balanced hormones, we rapidly develop diseases of aging, like hypertension, diabetes, arthritis, cancer, Alzheimer's, and heart disease.

But hormones are not just what keep us looking and feeling good when we are young; they are also huge determinants in what keeps us sexy, sexually active, and interested in having sex.

Throughout this book, you will find situations involving people whose hormones are out of balance. The results of these imbalances may include a lack or diminution of sex drive that may be totally out of proportion to what one would expect—or a sex drive that cannot be explained or correlated with the levels of hormones we see in blood tests. This is evidence that while hormones are crucial, they're only one of the many factors that determine the unique features of each person's sexuality, and evidence that our methods of measuring hormone levels are not reliable or reflective of any individual person's situation.

HUMAN AND NONHUMAN IDENTICAL HORMONES

Many women take hormones in various doses and formulations throughout their lifetimes, including birth control pills.

Women who take birth control pills often complain of loss of libido. Healthy women in their 20s and 30s—even those sexually active and in love with their partners—often confess they have little or no interest in sex. This is a sad situation that must be addressed, yet it is rarely discussed in the media or in medical journals. While researchers have reported on the negative effect of birth control pills on libido, little information about it reaches the women who are directly affected. When I see young women with loss of libido in good relationships, the first question I ask is, "Are you taking birth control pills?" If the answer is yes, we consider other options, and in most cases the woman goes off the pill and regains her sex drive in no time. Over the years I've prescribed my share of birth control pills. Yet I became disappointed and finally stopped prescribing them after watching too many young women unnecessarily robbed of their sexuality—sometimes leading to the loss of romantic relationships and marriages—as a direct result of these drugs.

Women's doctors owe their patients an honest explanation of the long-term consequences of taking the pill. Making sure all the side effects are understood and not brushed over is crucial before a woman is prescribed a drug she may take for the next 20 years of her life. Unfortunately, most physicians are as unaware of the problems associated with the pill as their patients, leading them to believe they are doing a service to women by continuing to prescribe them. Just note one more thing when you think of birth control pills. When doing blood tests to check hormone levels in women on birth control pills, we always find them to be at menopausal levels. That means the birth control pills have suppressed hormone production in young women so that the women may be 20, but their hormone levels are more like those of a 50-year-old woman, thus explaining the many side effects associated with their use. (See more about the pill's dark side on page 127.)

As women age, they have the option of taking hormone replacements in the form of either **human identical hormones** or **nonhuman identical hormones**. Studies on synthetic nonhuman identical hormones have demonstrated them to be less safe in older postmenopausal women than the hormone preparations known as **bioidentical hormones**. In fact, birth control pills and other synthetic hormones prescribed to women in menopause have similar side effects and problems. Bioidentical hormone preparations are prescription hormones, manufactured from soy and yam extracts through pharmaceutical processes of concentration and purification. Inside the body, they're recognized by cellular receptors as identical to the body's own hormones and are accepted by the body without negative reactions. Having the proper quantity and balance of hormones in the body is a great way to ensure optimal physiologic function, including a robust sex drive.

Unfortunately, fixing sexual problems isn't always as simple as balancing hormones. Another overwhelming and also little-discussed problem is that long-term relationships often become stale. Unless the partners actively work on keeping the sexual part of their relationship alive, passion leaves, attraction fades, and each partner's sexual desire for the other disappears as well. Even balanced hormones can't revive a dormant or dead love affair. As the stories of our lives unfold and sexuality progresses through the phases of our lives, change is the only guarantee. How we deal with the specific changes determines the outcomes of our lives and the evolution and survival of our sexuality. We'll talk about this in a lot more detail in later chapters.

Men, just like women, are directly affected by their hormones throughout their lives. Whether those hormones are made by their own bodies or taken in from the outside, they have a profound impact. Young men who use anabolic steroids to build muscles often experience unpleasant side effects. While these young men look buff and profess to be sexually charged, the truth may be different. Anabolic steroids in use since the 1930s—drugs like nandrolone, stanozolol, oxandrolone, and metandienone—are freely and naively used by teens and young men in gyms across the U.S.; they suppress normal testosterone production, causing the testicles to shrink, leaving many physically fit young men with an incongruously low sex drive. Over time, men using these substances end up feeling depleted and even depressed, along with experiencing other, often serious, short- and long-term consequences.[1]

REPORTED EFFECTS OF ANABOLIC STEROID USE MAY INCLUDE

- Psychiatric: aggressive behavior, hallucinations, depression, suicidal ideation
- Decreased testicular size
- Severe acne
- Balding
- Fluid retention
- Facial/chest hair in females
- Elevation of blood pressure and cholesterol
- Increased risk of heart attack
- Increased risk of cancer
- Spontaneous tendon rupture
- Sexual dysfunction, among other effects.[2]

Hormones are crucial in regulating and determining how our bodies and organs function; how we look; and, most importantly for our purpose, how we express ourselves as sexual beings. But what goes on in the body is directly connected to what goes on in the mind. And the person someone becomes psychologically as an adult is deeply shaped by the experiences of childhood.

PARENTAL GUIDANCE NECESSARY

This fact may make some people uncomfortable but none of us would be here if our parents didn't have sex! Even thinking about our parents' sex lives feels weird to most of us, but the truth is, how Mom and Dad related and possibly still do relate to each other sexually and in their relationship profoundly affects how people perceive love, intimacy, and sex as they enter their teen years and the next phases of their lives. Even if you weren't raised by your biological parents, how you saw them demonstrating affection or maybe avoiding showing you or your siblings their sexuality seeped into your subconscious. Your family of origin and their behavior, their connection to one another, and how you understood their relationship have a great deal to do with how you perceive and express your own sexuality as an adult. Your sexual spring, as I call it, includes the lessons about sex you witnessed as a child and how these lessons meld into the person you become as an adult.

When I talk to my patients about their childhood memories, I find a wide range of sexual role models in their past. At one extreme, are parents who were extremely sexual and physically demonstrative in front of others, including their children. At the other extreme, are parents who were cold and distant showing little emotion and affection toward each other or even their children. There are mothers and fathers who, after getting divorced or separated, became sexual with other partners to whom their children may have been exposed. Where you fall along this wide spectrum influences your own adult perception of intimacy and sex and even whether or not you make a connection between the two. You observed how the most important adults in your life—the people tasked with your very survival—related to one another, and those lessons sunk in whether you know it consciously or not.

Take a moment to think back to the attitudes surrounding sex and intimacy in your childhood home. Perhaps your parents condoned openly sexual behavior. Maybe they had an open marriage and you even knew their various partners. At the other extreme, you may have had parents who never brought up sex, or made it sound abnormal, dirty, and unacceptable and turned it into a taboo. Perhaps they subtly criticized your burgeoning. sexuality, or wouldn't let you date, or imposed unreasonable curfews. You might be the child of very young, or much older, parents. All these circumstances play into the way you come to view sexuality as an adult. Take some time and think back to your childhood home from the sexuality perspective and its connection to intimacy and affection. Your memories and conversations with siblings about their perception of your family home environment will help you better understand your attitude toward sex.

I want to share a few stories you may find useful and interesting, exemplifying the connection between upbringing and adult outcomes.

A male patient comes from a family with four boys. The parents were together for more than 50 years when the father died. My patient recalls in his early teens his mother would walk around the house in her underwear and ask for help hooking her bra from whichever son walked by. She talked about sex a lot too. When the boys got older and started to bring girlfriends around, the mother was flirtatious, more like a girlfriend than a mom. She would sit on the couch next to a son and put her head on his lap and talk to him in baby language. Many young women left after witnessing this strange mother–son relationship, perhaps fearing the mother wouldn't allow another woman in the sons' lives. The father never seemed to take notice of the strange relationship between the mother and sons. He was harsh and judgmental of the sons.

As they grew up, the boys—now men—had difficulty with intimate relationships. Most were withdrawn and unable to connect with women. It took decades of therapy for some of them to connect some of the problems they had with women may have come from their exposure to an overly sexual mother. Two of the brothers met women who understood them and helped them work things through, while the other two spent their entire lives confused in dysfunctional relationships. To this day, even though the mother has reached her 90s, she still focuses primarily on her sons ignoring their wives and their now adult children.

Another patient's mother had her in her teens. She left my patient to be raised by her grandmother, while the mother spent her life traveling around the world following various men who adored her at first and later spurned her. The grandmother was a wonderful woman who raised my patient wisely and caringly. My patient dedicated her life to helping others. Although she is highly evolved and intelligent, her personal life suffered from the mother's abandonment. She married a few times, but her fear of being abandoned—as her mother had done to her—stopped her short of having a fulfilling relationship with any one man.

A male friend is an only child of a post–World War II couple who lived through the hardships of life in a war-torn European country. Their son was their pride and joy, and while they came from humble beginnings and little formal education, they were committed to raising their son to be an educated man. Toward that end, the father spent long hours working far away from home and the son spent his entire childhood coddled by his lonely mother. When he was 12, the parents sent the boy to boarding school. The separation was hard on both mother and son. He barely graduated. As an adult, he made his life as far away as he could from his parents. He married a cold woman and had four kids he rarely saw, because his job, just like his father's, kept him away from his home. He never understood how to be intimate or share warmth and love. Sex was a simple act of de-stressing for this man. His children never learned to connect or be intimate either. The man became successful at work, but his personal life included a mixture of affairs and one-night stands.

And then there is the wonderful story of a friend whose parents set the example of a great loving and connected relationship. My friend and her brother were exposed to love, communication, and connection from the moment they woke up in the morning until they went to sleep at night. My friend married a wonderful man who adores her and is her perfect match. They have been married more than 30 years and have two great kids, and she and her husband still have a passionate love affair. When she entered menopause, she started taking hormones to support her vitality and libido, and she feels and looks as great now as she did when she was 35. One day her daughter told her she would only marry a man like her father. She did.

Finally, here is a story about childrearing in the 1990s in a suburb of New York City.

Years ago, when my younger daughter was in high school, the baseball team had a traditional annual party. The parties were held at different players' houses, and sometimes parents were present. This particular year, the party turned into a loud and raucous bash. Even though the kids were underage, alcohol flowed freely and they even had a stripper. Concerned neighbors called the police. The officers were shocked when the boy's parents opened the door! They were calm and relaxed, apparently indifferent to the drunken young boys and the naked stripper in their own home. The incident made the local papers, and legal action was taken against the parents.

But here's the strangest thing—almost no one besides the local authorities and the legal community thought there was anything wrong with the party! To this day, the parents of many of the other boys still say the authorities made a big deal over the episode and the only crime the boys' parents committed was that of getting caught. As the mother of teen girls at the time, I was sadly disappointed by the message these parents were sending. They were encouraging a totally disturbing trend. The most outrageous and sexually charged parties create popularity. Thus, boys and girls were learning to equate social success with drinking and reckless sexuality. This certainly was not the message I wanted to give my daughters.

Just look back at your own childhood and see what message your parents gave you. Then think some more and decide what message you want to give to your own children.

I have patients who complain how poorly their husbands treat them. They talk of having to put up with verbal and even physical abuse and fights that erode their own self-esteem and confidence. Women in these circumstances are rarely in the mood for sex, and often turn to their children for emotional support, shutting their husbands out. Whether these marriages ultimately dissolve or the couple gets help—or worse, continue the same destructive pattern into old age—the message they give their children is that it is okay for men to abuse women. They also give young women the message that they have no choice but to accept this situation. Sadly, a large number of children end up following in their parents' footsteps. Only some will go to extremes to radically change their own situations from what they saw at home.

A child of one such toxic marriage is Sandy, a patient in her early 20s. Sandy is an extremely bright, beautiful woman who unfortunately wastes much of her intellect dreaming up ways to manipulate her divorced parents into giving her money, which she usually spends on clothes, clubs, alcohol, and drugs. She told me she likes to "party" with older men, whom she invariably has sex with. She constantly finds herself discarded when the novelty of hooking up with a "wild child" wears off. Sandy's mother, June, also a patient, is a successful professional who focused on getting her life together after her husband left her for a woman 30 years her junior. Before that Sandy watched June quietly suffering through her husband's blatant cheating for more than a decade. June believes her daughter will outgrow her current phase and stop allowing men to mistreat her because June herself moved on with her own life and set a good example for her daughter. That may not be enough for Sandy, though. She spent 10 of her formative years watching her father abuse her mother. Just because June has moved on doesn't mean Sandy can or will. My advice to June has been to stop giving Sandy money unless it goes specifically toward therapy. While June is now living her life happily, Sandy doesn't have the tools to make the right choices in her life. She needs professional help.

Another one of my patients, Claire, is almost 40 and never married, despite a long line of boyfriends. She is desperate to find a life partner and start a family, but her parents set a really tough example she can't get out of her head. When she was a teen, she saw her father in a restaurant holding hands with a woman who wasn't her mother. She ran home and told her mother, who responded by calmly telling her she knew the father was having an affair. After disclosing that bombshell to her impressionable teen daughter, the mother went on as if nothing happened and never mentioned the affair again—neither to her husband nor her children. Everything was swept under the rug, and life in Claire's childhood home continued as if nothing was wrong. Her parents are now in their 80s and still married, and her mother continues to act as though they have a perfect marriage. Every time Claire has tried to speak to her mother about the husband's infidelity, she hit a brick wall. Claire spent decades on a therapist's couch. Loyalty, trust, intimacy, and sex are confused in her mind, and fear rules her personal relationships. She still doesn't trust her own judgment and consistently chooses boyfriends who are unfaithful or unreliable, or just finds herself in abusive and destructive situations with men. Perhaps not surprisingly, Claire's brother grew up to be a womanizer who treats women abominably. Despite therapy, Claire's life is still difficult and confusing. I hope Claire finds her self-confidence and, along with it, the right man finally arrives. A man who does not resemble her father, so she doesn't have to continue living in fear of becoming her mother.

WHERE IN THE WORLD?

Uptight New England Yankee? Sultry Southern belle? Free-wheeling California girl? These may be stereotypes, but where in America—or in the world—you were raised also has an important impact on your sexuality and your ability to be intimate. America has always been a melting pot, and the influences of the countries from which parents and grandparents emigrated figure strongly in the mix. There are cultures both within and outside of the United States where girls must remain virgins until they marry. In these cultures, sex must be only about procreation and only with one partner—the husband. It is not for enjoyment or frivolous fun. There are other societies that encourage freedom of expression and choice when it comes to marriage, love, and sex. Some social groups frown on divorce. For others, it's practically a rite of passage. One thing cuts across all social groups, however; most Western societies romanticize couples, and not being part of one is regarded as abnormal or a sign of failure. All these influences shape our beliefs about what sex should—and shouldn't—be.

Beyond how your parents or guardians acted, there are other factors that affected you and led to your choices and perspective on sex. What kinds of books and magazines were in your home when you were growing up? What movies were you allowed or forbidden to watch? Were opinions about sex positive and open or negative and hidden, a constant source of criticism? I have a patient who was a teenager in the 1980s. Her mother used to forbid her from listening to Madonna's music, because she thought Madonna was too slutty, too sexual. Meanwhile, many of my patient's friends dressed like Madonna trying to emulate her "bad girl" persona. What your parents say and do leave indelible marks on you. This young woman was caught between her mother and her friends. She chose her friends, and the next two decades became a sex frenzy for her. She became the bad girl because she hated her mother's rigidity and did everything to fight it. In the process, she got hurt. Her self-esteem was so low she allowed men to abuse her, and she lived a destructive and promiscuous life for many years.

When my younger daughter was around 12, we went clothes shopping with one of her friends and the friend's mother. At the time the girls were starting to develop breast buds, the first blush of puberty. The friend's mother was a pretty woman who acted much younger than her age and had a great body that she dressed to show. As our girls started trying on tween-sexy clothes, moving into the next stage of their lives, I noticed the friend's mother trying on some of the same clothes her daughter was trying. I took her aside and gently pointed out it was our girls' time and the focus should be on them, not on us. She and I could go shopping anytime, but on that trip we needed to get out of the way so our girls could start to feel good about their own new looks. A light bulb seemed to go off in her head as she listened, and she quickly let her daughter take center stage. I believe that her mature and caring behavior contributed to steering her daughter onto the road of great self-confidence. Today, that little girl is a highly successful college professor, happily married to a wonderful man who adores and respects her.

Being the parent of a girl in our overly sexualized culture involves toeing a fine line between providing serious boundaries and allowing room to find her own identity and the freedom to express it. I'll go into more about this in the next chapter. In my practice, I hear from parents going to extremes trying to ban sexy clothes and control sexual interactions of any kind, such as books and pictures and even access to the internet. I believe in boundaries, and in protecting our kids from harm. But we have to remember that our young girls don't always understand the implications or consequences of a short skirt or a revealing top. To them, they're just following what's "in." As parents, we have to learn to guide our girls—by example, and by reining them in and guiding them to smart choices—without extreme limitations or harsh bans. In my experience, the parents who rigidly set limits without communicating clearly and openly with their children about why they disapprove of an outfit or an action often send their kids spinning into outright rebellion. It's extremely important to be present when talking with your daughter, even if just for 10 minutes a day. Honesty and kindness, listening to the teen and setting fair boundaries lead to outstanding outcomes.

And what about you? Think about the messages you received while growing up. Whether they were subliminal or in-your-face, you absorbed those sexual opinions, how sex and intimacy were or weren't connected, which in turn helped you form your own views. And think about all the people you met throughout your growing years: teachers, friends, relatives, and neighbors. All, in their own way, had an impact on you.

FAITH OF OUR FATHERS—AND MOTHERS

My patients come from a wide variety of backgrounds. In terms of religion, their families range from nonbelievers to those who observe significant holidays, to those who go to church every Sunday, followers of rules and rituals. From a historical perspective, religions create rules and guidelines for behavior. Very clear rules of engagement for sexual behavior make up a significant part of many religious systems.

Perhaps you've seen the movie *Carrie*, in which a repressed, religious-fanatic mother condemns her daughter simply for getting her period. I actually have a patient with such a background. Evelyn, in her 30s, came from a very religious family in which all talk of sex was absolutely forbidden. Her mother told her that having a period made her dirty and that being interested in sex was only acceptable for prostitutes. Not only has Evelyn never married, she never had sex. She says that she thinks she may prefer women to men but has yet to experience a sexual or romantic relationship with either gender. A good Samaritan who spends her entire life helping others with kindness and love, she reminds me of Mother Teresa. She cares for everyone, and her identity is tied entirely into service to others.

Another patient is Maribel, in her 60s, who also came from a very religious family. Her parents admonished her of the non-negotiable importance of marrying a man of her own faith. But love had a way of its own. When she was in her early 20s, Maribel fell in love with a man of a different religion. Her parents threatened to disown her if she married him. She was devastated, but in the end respected their wishes and broke off the relationship. She never went out with another man, choosing instead to immerse herself into her career. In the end, her mother—in her 80s—admitted that her family's rigidity not only deprived her of grandchildren but may have ruined her daughter's emotional life as well. To this day Maribel never talks about sex or romance. If someone brings the subject up, she immediately disconnects.

And then there is Julie, a young woman from a very strict family who was forbidden to even interact with anyone outside their faith. Her religion keeps everyone in tightly knit clusters, allowing little exposure to the outside world. When she turned 16, she ran away from home to New York City and became a waitress. Her family disowned her and told everyone in the community she was dead. They even held a funeral for her!

Julie spent years heavy into drugs—heroin, crack cocaine—and alcohol.

After 10 years, Julie took charge of her life and decided to live the best version of her life possible. She joined an AA group and read many self-help books. In time she gained her self-confidence, became sober and redirected her life to focus on joy, self-kindness and positivity. A few years later she met a man of a different faith but with similar philosophical beliefs—whom she married—went back to school, and together they built a solid and happy family. As a social worker, she now finds fulfillment helping other women escape oppressive environments, and she is happily married with children she is raising very differently than she was raised. Julie is spiritual. She tells me she respects her background and she appreciates what she learned in her parents' home. However, she found her own way, and while she isn't religious, she is raising her kids to develop insight and kindness while giving them more freedom than she had. Her children are now young teens and thriving while Julie and her husband seem to have a solid relationship. Intimacy is what they both believe is at the core of their relationship, and they have sex on a regular basis too. They both strongly believe sex connects them and keeps them intimate.

YOU CAN'T ESCAPE THE MEDIA

Unless you have moved to an isolated mountaintop and are reading this book by candlelight, you are probably like the rest of us—constantly being bombarded with messages about sexuality from the media, Internet, and through art, sports, entertainment, and advertising. Headlines about celebrity hook-ups and royal weddings abound; we're inundated with gossip about who's in and who's out of the homosexual closet and which politician and media mogul is harassing and molesting women. Fashion magazines reinforce that we don't have the bodies to dress like the celebrities we deify or have their sex appeal; most of the supermodels we idolatrize seem to be 15, size zero, and flat-chested, with their images fully Photoshopped. No wonder none of the clothes they sport ever look good on a normal size-12 woman with breasts and hips.

Advertisements tell women they must dye their hair and wear makeup to be attractive. Advice on how to dress and smell and look to be sexier is coupled with advice on how to achieve the perfect orgasm and how to attract and please our partners. In between, we're reading tell-all memoirs, listening to explicit music, and watching highly sexualized music videos. It seems the entire world around us is pushing the idea that sex is everywhere, and it had better be the most important thing on our priority list or we are abnormal and missing out on the most important thing in life.

Nowhere is this more apparent than in ads for erectile dysfunction. Look at the gauzy lighting, the gentle music, the athletic, gray-haired man walking hand in hand through the autumn leaves with his lovely, slightly younger wife. Note that the underlying cause of the problem is really poor blood flow everywhere in the body due to atherosclerotic thickening of the arteries. That's just what happens with age. One of the ways we can see this is in the case of erectile dysfunction, but also in strokes and heart attacks, which just happen to be potentially fatal conditions. Interestingly, this very important fact and the potential side effects of the medication are not mentioned until the end of the commercial—you know, that segment when the announcer's voice suddenly becomes very soft, almost unintelligible, and sounds like it's on fast-forward. Even though the problem is caused by the impaired blood flow to the penis due to atherosclerosis, not lack of Viagra, that inconvenient fact is never mentioned. Instead, the commercial focuses on creating the illusion that sex should always happen "when the moment strikes" and of course the man "must be ready". What about the women? How do they feel about erectile dysfunction or the "perfect moment"? No one knows, because they, like the men in these ridiculous commercials, never speak. The pharmaceutical manufacturers don't show us real people like you and me. They prefer to influence us subliminally, with good-looking actors smiling as if they've just had the best sex of their lives. No wonder we believe that unless we have sex regardless of our age, we are not okay.

This Hollywood hedonistic vision of sexuality reinforces the fantasy that once people get together, sex, intimacy, and love will just automatically follow, leading to a beautiful, sexy, fulfilling "forever after." It's a lovely idea, but it may not be the whole truth. The fact that sex may not always be the most important part of a relationship is rarely if ever mentioned. I can't tell you the number of patients who've whispered to me, "It seems like the whole world is having amazing sex, and I'm the only one who isn't. What am I doing wrong? What's wrong with me? Can you please fix me so I can be like everyone else?" The people who ask me are men, women, and transgender people; old and young; single and married; straight, gay, lesbian, and bisexual; yet all seem to believe that everyone else was handed the key to unlock the secrets of sex and intimacy, and they alone were left out in the cold.

My patients tell me that when sex leaves their lives, they feel like utter failures because they are not living up to the impossible standard reflected in media images around them every single day. Embarrassed to admit this, they feel alone and are often loneliest in their closest relationships. More than a few of my patients have confided that they lie to their friends and family about their sex lives.

"Everyone else is having sex, but we aren't," is another statement I've heard countless times. Some go on to say that while they know that books, television shows, and movies don't depict real people, and that characters are idealized, they still want to be like those characters. Who wouldn't, when these men and women are often made to appear to be at the peak of their good looks and we are so desperately tempted to believe they know what's right for us far better than we do? Armies of art directors, costume designers, hair and makeup people, and gifted cinematographers see to it that the stars you watch onscreen always ooze sex and vitality. As a result, most of us set our sights on becoming just like these dream people, whose relationships and even appearance may just be pure fiction. To keep up the facade, we often tell others that our sex lives are terrific, even when they are far from it.

If we want to live genuine, happier, and less stressful lives, it's time to put this fairy tale to rest, face what is really going on, and change it if we really believe it needs fixing. Hormones can make a big difference, but there is one absolute requirement for creating, maintaining, and rekindling lifelong sexuality: an honest, connected, committed, intimate, real relationship.

One of my patients, Martha, is in her late 60s and retired. Skinny, with long gray hair, she suffered numerous accidents that led to multiple surgeries. She appears frail and sometimes acts her age, although the hormone regimen I've created for her has helped restore much of her vitality. She has been married for many decades, often talks with much love for her husband, and swears that they still enjoy sex at least twice a week. They frequently travel and enjoy each other's company. She says sex keeps their relationship youthful and keeps their life together exciting. They are passionate about each other and are both interested and interesting. Intimacy has never gone missing in their relationship, and neither has sex. I believe her.

I *don't* believe Shelley, a well to do glamorous socialite in her 50s on hormones since she started having symptoms of menopause in her late 40s. Shelley practically lives at the plastic surgeon's office, has gorgeous hair extensions, wears the trendiest designer clothes, and shows off her gym-toned tan body. She tells me she has sex with her husband of 35 years four times a week. He is a man in a very powerful position, and comes from a culture that condones men having sex outside the marriage.

Shelley wants everyone to believe she and her husband are the perfect couple and that he never strays because she keeps him sexually satisfied. He travels extensively and spends large chunks of time away from home. To me, it appears she's trying too hard to convince others that her life is perfect, and I think it's more about convincing herself. Who cares if her sex life with her husband isn't perfect? Shelley is a wonderful woman in her own right. She is a contributor to society in so many ways, she writes and publishes books and articles, and she contributes to many charities. It's sad to think she defines herself as the wife who will do anything to stay young-looking, sexual and desirable, making sexuality the defining factor in her life.

And then there are some people, too discouraged to fight the discrimination permeating our age-obsessed culture, just give up. I was at a party where a divorced woman in her late 50s sadly told everyone who would listen that "once you are fifty, it's all over. You can't wear strapless dresses or plunging neck-lines. *You're not sexy anymore.* And not only are you not sexy, you might as well not even exist. That's how I used to look at women our age when I was in my 20s and 30s, and now I am one of those old women."

Many women her age—and older—loudly disagreed, some saying they still had active, rewarding, sexually intimate relation-ships, but she pushed back: "You're all wrong. If anyone actually says they are still having sex at my age, they're lying. There is no room for sex as you get older. I would never take my clothes off in front of a man. Do you really think a man wants to see my wrinkled body? I don't think so. In fact, I wish all women our age would just get out of the way and give up on this crazy notion that we can keep up with the younger ones. Just seeing young women reminds me how horrible I look. Aging is tough, and there are no options."

This poor woman, feeling so terrible about herself is a sad and negative model for other women in her age group. Depressed and unwilling to take any steps toward coming to terms with her age and building a happier life for herself, she has instead decided to keep her heart closed to possibly meeting a man, having convinced herself that her age precludes a positive outcome. She is not uncommon among many older women who become victims of our youth-obsessed culture. I feel sorry for her, and I am sure if she were less angry and self-critical, her life would be much better. I'm not saying an attitude make-over would bring Prince Charming to her door, but I believe her life would be less frustrating and sad if she accepted aging as a normal part of life without focusing exclusively on its negative aspects and the perceived need for a man to make her life better. She has experience and wisdom, after all. Those are really sexy traits, and I often see young men with older women who don't seem to see the wrinkles.

I don't want to minimize that it's a hard world out there. As we search for our sexual identity at all ages, the only thing we can count on is change. We are at the mercy of our hormones, our parents' expectations, religious and cultural mores, and the ubiquitous media with its portrayals of "reality," leading us to believe we must be sexually active 24/7 and stay 25 regardless of chronologic age. Reality is different and if we want to enjoy our lives we must make it work. Over the course of three to five decades, we all lose the hormone-driven sexuality of youth—but that doesn't mean we have to lose our identity and positive outlook as individuals.

Sexuality and intimacy are defined by an infinite number of variables and elements. While "intimacy" has the same meaning regardless of age, the meaning of "sexuality" changes over the course of our lives and is unique to each one of us. In the next chapters, we'll explore how to find and define our personal identities in the sea of influences on our lives.

CHAPTER 3

TEEN SPIRIT: HORMONES GONE WILD

"Teenagers are like atoms when they're moving at hundreds of miles an hour and bouncing off each other."
—Anton Yelchin

You may recall what it was like. That feeling of expectation. Of unlimited possibility. The flush in your face. The pounding of your heart. Butterflies in your stomach. The twinges and pulses in parts of your body you never knew existed. We all lived through those tumultuous years and surprisingly, most of us even made it to adulthood. Some of us think back on those years with wistful nostalgia, while others are grateful just to have survived them. Teen years are the true spring of our sexuality, the years when our bodies first blossom and turn us from innocent children into naive yet sexually charged beings.

It's crucial to understand the profound impact hormonal changes have on teen bodies and minds.

Let's start with children. Before puberty, boys and girls are physiologically quite similar. The question of the impact of nature versus nurture on gender has been studied by researchers in many fields: anthropology, sociology, biology, and psychology. While certain gender-specific behaviors may be inborn, certain drugs and in utero (womb) hormones affect gender. The way children are raised in their particular cultures, communities and families count strongly into how they express their "boyness" or "girlness" to the outside world. As children enter puberty, sex hormones burst onto the scene. That leads to dramatic changes in the way teen bodies develop, leading to striking changes and differences on the outside and on the inside.

Difficult, challenging, exciting. As early as age nine or 10 up to 19 or even the early 20s, adolescents' bodies undergo momentous changes. Often the changes are difficult emotional and mental transformations. Perhaps the most obvious and most frequently focused-on transformation revolves around sexuality and the thoughts and actions sexuality generates in the young adult. Teens change under the influence of their new internal environment that is now ruled by the production of estrogen, progesterone, and testosterone. Sex hormones suddenly turn a playful child into a sexual being. Interest in sex soars as sex hormones flood the system and rule decisions and actions.

HORMONES RUN THE SHOW

A problem with teens is that sex hormones kick into high gear long before they have the maturity, life experiences, and wisdom to make sense of the myriad conflicting emotions they experience. Their sexuality and often sudden and seemingly inexplicable changes in behavior are initially hormone-fueled. With the onset of puberty and the hormonally induced sexual awakening, physical changes and sexuality take precedence over prior experience and emotional maturity. Girls and some boys at this stage may become obsessed with romance, hearts, and flowers, but for the most part, these fantasies are often cultural masks for the major motivator brought on by the arrival of hormones on the scene—the desire to have sex.

Teens are at a crossroads, propelled by their bodies into sexual situations they barely comprehend. Lacking a road map for sexual behavior, they follow their peers, media, and their parents' example. When my daughters were teens, I found myself in a constant dilemma, caught between the example I tried to set at home and the relentless pressures surrounding them from friends and the outside world—especially social media. Make no mistake about it—selling sexually laden content to teens is a very lucrative business. Ruthless people encourage naive teens to follow the examples of young and reckless celebrities who drink too much, take drugs, party too much, have indiscriminate sex, and wind up in rehab—too often portrayed as a badge of honor to their fans. Glossy magazines, gossip sites, social media, and music videos glorify and encourage overt sexuality and invariably associate it with bad behavior, and it is very difficult for even the most committed parents to counteract and balance out these influences.

As a mom, I tried to keep up as much as I could with the influx of media raining down on my girls, so I'd have the correct information and understanding of their teen world to provide balance and support for them. It's unrealistic to attempt to know everything your kids are exposed to, or to be able to control the limitless impact that social media and friends have on your child. But that does not mean modern parents should abdicate their involvement with and responsibility for their teens and deny what their kids are up to—leaving the teen vulnerable to dangerous behavior.

Recently, I was in Toronto, giving a daylong seminar to doctors on how to use bioidentical hormones in disease prevention and wellness. As we discussed the role of hormones at all stages of the life cycle, the topic of teen sexuality came up, as it invariably does when people speak of hormones at different ages. Most of the doctors in the audience were parents of teens, with professional and personal interest in the conversation.

After we discussed the science behind hormones in teenagers, I expressed my opinion that, left unchecked, sexual desire—lust—can become the sole driver of teen behavior, despite potential undesirable and dangerous consequences. As an example, I mentioned the phenomenon of "rainbow parties." My audience looked at me blankly. I was surprised how few of the parents in the room had heard about them, despite the fact they seem to be a common albeit disputed fad with teens in middle school.[1]

Boredom, the desire to be popular with peers, and the forces of social media are the reason rainbow parties exist. Actually, I'd say "desperation parties" is a far more accurate term to describe them, at least in the case of the girls who participate. If you, like the doctors in my seminar, don't know what a rainbow party is, then take a deep breath while I explain. First, a parent-free location is found and then advertised via Facebook and other social media to the teens in the group. Young girls, seeking the holy grail of teen popularity, each put on a different shade of lipstick, and then sequentially perform oral sex on the boys at the party. The boy with the largest array of lipstick colors on his penis is deemed the most popular.

I shared with my audience the story of Chelsea, a 15-year-old patient: quick-witted, with pretty brown eyes, slightly overweight. Chelsea confided in me that she sadly wasn't in the popular crowd at her school—calling her personal clique of friends "the B-list." The A-list girls, she said, were all pretty, mostly blonde with long hair, and very thin. So when she was unexpectedly invited to a rainbow party, she couldn't have been more flattered and excited about the possibility of finally fitting in with the cool kids. The day of the party, she spent hours at the mall, trying to find the brightest, shiniest lipstick. She extensively researched oral sex techniques and even practiced on a banana. Needless to say, she performed well. The boys—even the sports stars, the highest-ranked boys on the desirability scale—noticed her. She came to my office and described the experience in detail.

I had been working with her for six months at that point and she had lost a decent amount of weight, yet I had never seen her so animated and happy. More invitations to these parties followed, and on those party nights, she told me she thought herself the most popular girl in the room. She no longer felt like a loser, she proudly reported, because after her performances all the boys paid attention to her now.

The medical professionals I shared this story with were stunned. The ones who had daughters were totally sure their girls would never be part of such a thing. Maybe they were right. Maybe they wished they hadn't heard the story. In any case, the point was to raise parents' awareness that teens will get involved in potentially dangerous behavior as they have little experience or common sense driven primarily by their budding sexuality and peer pressure. Parents rarely know everything their kids are up to, and even if they believe their teens would never engage in risky behavior, someone's teen is. Unless individual teens proactively decide they do not belong in that kind of environment, they are prey to bad advice and bad company. So it behooves parents to be alert and help their teens channel their sexual energy into safer activities. Of course, sexual energy can be channeled into other pursuits. Some teens may turn into serious hard-working students while others may turn to religion or volunteering, athletic endeavors, video games or afterschool activities. Depending on the involvement of parents and the cultural, religious, and socioeconomic environment, teens' biological drives will play out differently.

And don't discount those cultural influences. Teens are constantly inundated with the antics of their media-appointed so-called role models—with lifestyles that embrace promiscuity, drugs, breaking the law, and the abuse of women. It's difficult to predict which way your teen will turn, but the outcome hinges on your relationship with your kid and his or her evolving self. This includes building his or her self-confidence, your steadfast presence, and your ability to listen to and validate your child as a separate person from you.

Where boys are concerned, many parents I meet professionally and socially seem less worried about potential promiscuity than about getting a girl pregnant. In fact, indiscriminate sex is too often not-so-silently accepted as a teenage boy's birthright. The dangerous "boys will be boys" attitude has been the impetus behind several prominent date- and gang-rape stories in the news. That's not surprising, given the behavior of many teenagers' sports and celebrity role models. This puts an unfair and difficult onus on the girls. That is why parents need to stay involved and provide solid role models. When parents don't actively participate in leveling the playing field of teen sexuality, they only perpetuate an adult culture of sexism, inequality, and confused priorities.

In today's teen culture, boys and girls still follow different rules and roles, pretty much the same as they always have. For most teen girls, being defined as someone's girlfriend is sadly a more important status symbol than earning a place in the National Honor Society. Athletes, especially football players, are usually the most sought-after, and girls may do practically anything to date a football star. For too many parents, it's more difficult to confront issues head-on than to ignore them. Unfortunately, if issues are ignored, the problems worsen as the teen gets older.

What's the result here? A massive lack of self-esteem for the girls that too often will continue into their 20s and beyond. Too many smart, talented young women intentionally derail themselves from academic, artistic, or athletic pursuits solely to become popular. Traumatic experiences of teen years are difficult to recover from. For boys who participate in these scenarios the explicit message that girls—and women—are expected to maintain subservient roles is reinforced. If respect for girls and women is not taught to boys while they're young, they don't have the incentive to develop boundaries for their sexuality or respect for women. If they do not get the example of mutual respect at home, it is more difficult for them to develop successful intimate relationships as adults.

Of course, not all teenagers act this way. Many learn about emotional growth and real relationships from their teachers, spiritual leaders, mentors, and parents. Many of these young men go on to become responsible adults motivated by respect and kindness, setting great examples for their partners, peers and, eventually, their own children.

Yet even the lucky girls with good support and caring parents have another stumbling block facing them. The blanketing of America, including its teens, with birth control pills leads to more problems than solutions. The misperception of what birth control pills represent directly affects both sexuality and actions.

QUESTIONING THE PILL

One of the many reasons teen girls engage in sex so easily without thinking about consequences is the implicit encouragement they receive from our medical profession. Over the past four decades, I've watched with increasing disappointment as the American College of Obstetrics and Gynecology—the leading ob-gyn society—has climbed on the bandwagon of mass-prescribing birth control pills for teenage girls to regulate their periods and eliminate acne, as well as for as the FDA-approved use—preventing pregnancy. I have no doubt that all mothers who take their daughters to the gynecologist to get them started on the pill believe they are doing a wise, well-informed, safe, and protective, practical thing.

Physicians don't explain why they give birth control pills so freely to young girls. Many mothers tell me gynecologists and even primary care physicians routinely give their 12–15-year-old girls birth control pills for irregular periods or acne. The FDA has not approved the use of the pill as a way to regulate periods. In fact, there are no studies demonstrating the health benefits of regular periods in teens. Very few physicians know the implications of giving birth control pills so freely. Even if they do, there is such a big push to use them that few go against the tide and risk losing patients or being reprimanded by their peers and medical societies. As for the mothers, by sanctioning the possibility of consequence-free use of birth control pills, they are not only agreeing that it's okay to have sex, they are encouraging it.

Reliable studies have indicated that abstinence-only sex education doesn't work,[2] so many mothers go along with the use of birth control pills, assuming that teenagers will have sex no matter what. Mothers mean well, and protecting their daughters against unplanned pregnancy does make sense, but it doesn't address the crucial health issue of sexually transmitted diseases (STDs) and the long-term side effects of birth control pills. Prescribing birth control pills freely and leading teens to believe there are no consequences add to the emotional and social pressures heaped on girls, implicitly pushes them to define their self-worth on the basis of their sexual attractiveness and popularity. Also, by giving birth control pills to girls, boys do not have to take responsibility in the act.

As I was raising my daughters and they entered puberty and adolescence, I did my best to be at home and accessible even more than during their younger years, so we could address issues of sexuality, popularity, and self-esteem. To me, keeping my daughters feeling safe and grounded and putting a premium on high self-esteem were the keys to raising successful adults who would not equate male sexual attention and having sex to their self-worth.

Neither one of my daughters took birth control pills. I strongly suggested they use condoms for their safety and they listened. Almost all their friends were taking birth control pills by the time they were 14. Most of their physicians did not address concern for safety, impact of sexual behavior, STDs, sex and intimacy. Personally, I think the ubiquitous use of birth control pills is an invitation to reckless lifestyles and increases the danger of sexually transmitted diseases; in fact, it has led to disenfranchising women instead of empowering them. (Using birth control pills as a public health tool for women and girls in parts of the world without access to healthcare or education is not the same as indiscriminately prescribing them to young women who have consistent access to medical care and education, and who also have other choices for their reproductive health.)

One thing the pill doesn't do is protect against STDs. While some sexually transmitted diseases are easily treated with antibiotics, there are some that are dangerous and even deadly. Why isn't that message getting to parents and their daughters? What kind of empowerment are we producing when we jeopardize our children's lives? And even if an antibiotic or a vaccine can treat or prevent long term consequences of some STDs, why are we accepting this as a solution rather than stressing prevention through education and empowerment? Viruses like herpes, human papilloma virus (HPV), and human immunodeficiency virus (HIV) are particularly well known, dangerous, and often incurable.[3] They are permanent life-changers for young people at risk who don't understand or know their impact until decades later.

HUMAN PAPILLOMA VIRUS (HPV)

HPV is a sexually transmitted viral infection. Also known as venereal warts, it includes more than 100 types of viruses. The problem is that while 90 percent of these viruses resolve like the common cold, by themselves, around 10 percent may not. There are a few strains that are associated with an increased risk of cervical cancer. It takes decades for the HPV strains that are dangerous to become cancers, and women who have regular Pap smears have at least a 99 percent chance of preventing this type of cancer. HPV has also been linked to pelvic inflammatory disease (PID) and infertility, along with other sexually transmitted diseases like gonorrhea, chlamydia, and other bacterial infections. A vaccine has been developed to decrease the risk associated with some of the most virulent HPV strains. While this vaccine may be a good public health tool, it still begs the question of safety for the individual. There are also many rarely discussed side effects that should give a mother pause when deciding whether to give her nine-year-old daughter or son the vaccine.[4]

The public interest group Judicial Watch reported 371 serious adverse events in patients who received Merck's HPV vaccine Gardasil, including three deaths. The aggressively marketed vaccine comes with reports of serious adverse reactions, including anaphylaxis, a serious allergic reaction that may cause death. Other reactions have included disorders of the blood and lymphatic systems as well as of the respiratory, gastrointestinal, immune, musculoskeletal, nervous, and vascular systems.[5]

As of May 31, 2017, it is noteworthy that 57,520 vaccine reaction reports were made to the Federal Vaccine Adverse Reporting Systems including 271 deaths from Gardasil and all other HPV vaccines (VAERS).[6]

One girl died of a blood clot three hours after receiving the vaccine. A 19-year-old died of heart failure partially caused by large blood clots two weeks after getting the vaccine. According to the Centers for Disease Control and Prevention, both patients were taking birth control pills that raise the risk of blot clots, thus adding another dangerous side effect to this cocktail. A 12-year-old died of heart complications six days after receiving Gardasil, according to VAERS reports.

The label on Gardasil states that it should not be given to pregnant women, and 18 of 42 pregnant women who were given Gardasil experienced adverse side effects, ranging from spontaneous abortion to fetal abnormalities. Clinical trials used in the FDA's review of Gardasil last year showed five cases of birth defects among women who received the vaccine within 30 days of conception.[7]

In February 2007, when Gardasil came on the market, I wrote on my blog (www.drerika.com): "The HPV vaccine has only been tested for fewer than five years on possibly as few as 10,000 10-year-old girls in Africa. No one knows what will happen to those girls or our girls in five, 10, or 20 years after the vaccine has been administered. The only science here is the real live testing about to be done on our daughters, who are technically, like the African 10-year-olds, guinea pigs. Remember the Lyme vaccine? What happened to that cure-all?[8] It killed a few people and was quickly off the market."[9]

While I and many others in the medical community were speaking out and sounding the alarm, Merck was investing hundreds of millions of dollars into lobbying and marketing the vaccine, and initially succeeded in persuading the governor of Texas to mandate its use on sixth-grade schoolgirls. Only a revolt by parents and community groups put a stop to that situation. The pharmaceutical giant recently submitted another supplemental biological license application to the FDA to market Gardasil to prevent vaginal and vulvar cancers. And Merck's influence has only grown as the years have passed. While initially recommended exclusively and specifically to young girls who were not yet sexually active, Gardasil has been rereleased and is now marketed to sexually active women of all ages as well as boys and men. The real truth about its use—and usefulness—remains in question. Pediatricians who receive all their information from the drug rep intimidate and bully mothers into having their daughters and now sons immunized in spite of questionable outcomes from the vaccine. The end of the HPV vaccine story has not been written yet.

The question remains: Do we need a vaccine like Gardasil, or would we be better off providing real support and education to our teens to help them lead safer and more empowered lives? Isn't prevention the best medicine?

HUMAN IMMUNODEFICIENCY VIRUS (HIV)

HIV, the virus that causes AIDS in its active disease form, is primarily a sexually transmitted virus that has gone from being a death sentence to being a serious and expensive but treatable chronic disease. The CDC has proved itself worthy of praise with the discovery and development of a cocktail of medications that has saved the lives of hundreds of thousands of the afflicted; people positive for HIV were dying by the thousands in the 1980s and 1990s before this treatment became available. However, the treatment is very expensive and not without serious side effects. HIV, which initially carried a serious social stigma, is more common in gay men and drug users, who may be more unlikely to get good medical care or practice safe sex. The virus is transmitted via bodily fluids, meaning primarily through sexual contact without protection. A carrier of HIV can transmit the HIV virus through sexual contact and thus spread the disease.

While much progress has been made, HIV is still life-changing and life-threatening. Prevention by teaching and encouraging safe sex, helping diminish promiscuous sexual behavior and intravenous drug usage, is the key to keeping young men and women safe. This is a public health issue that must be treated with constant vigilance and with the clear understanding that HIV and its active disease, AIDS, affect not just the infected individual but also entire families and the fabric of our society.[10]

TEEN SEX: STATISTICS FROM THE FRONT LINES

According to the Centers for Disease Control and Prevention, it really is a jungle out there when it comes to teen sexuality. This is serious business.

A 2011 survey of U.S. high school students[11] found that:

- 47.4 percent had had sexual intercourse
- 33.7 percent had had sexual intercourse during the previous three months, and of these, 39.8 percent did not use a condom the last time they had sex
- 76.7 percent did not use birth control in any form to prevent pregnancy the last time they had sex
- 15.3 percent had had sex with four or more people during their high school years

In other studies:

- In the 40 US states reporting to CDC, an estimated 8,300 people, ages 13 to 24, had an HIV infection in 2009[12]
- Nearly half of the 19 million new STDs each year are among people ages 15 to 24 years[13]

TEENS RUN WILD

At a seminar I was teaching in New York City, the issue of birth control pills came up. A gynecologist in the audience, genuinely caring and interested in helping young women, asked if there were safer methods than birth control pills that we could offer our young women to protect them from sexually transmitted diseases and unwanted pregnancies, while still encouraging them to feel free and empowered. A lengthy discussion ensued between the participating physicians, some of whom were parents as well as gynecologists and primary care practitioners. As physicians, we all hope to help steer our society to healthier shores, yet we are limited by the tools we have and the information we possess.

Sadly, the best we could do at that seminar was face headfirst the sobering fact that the birth control pill train left the station long ago. Birth control pills are promoted as the perfect example of empowerment for women, while the true picture isn't quite so glorious. Birth control pills may allow women to feel free sexually because they eliminate the monthly fear of getting pregnant, but they don't prevent sexually transmitted diseases, they don't encourage intimate relationships and mutual respect, they don't really empower women, and their dangers may outweigh their benefits.

So how are we helping our young girls? How are we protecting them? We aren't really. We just throw them into the water without teaching them how to swim or giving them a useful life vest. Sexuality and promiscuity in teens are too closely connected, and neither parents nor teens really know—or want to know—how to minimize the danger.

Parents want to believe that their teens don't have sex, but the hard truth is that many of them do. Mothers and fathers must take responsibility for supervising their kids. When a daughter leaves the house wearing too short a skirt, too tight a top, or too revealing an outfit, a parent must speak up. Honest discussions about the messages your teen is sending to their world, as well as the possible consequences of those messages, are just part of good parenting. Most teens want to be cool and dress like their peers and their celebrity role models. Self-expression is important, but if parents won't give them an adult and experienced perspective on the possible consequences of their actions, who will? While it's true that teens find lots of ways of getting around restrictions, talking to them about sex is essential to providing them with support and real parenting. Too many teenage girls in my practice describe examples of meager and unsuccessful attempts at parental guidance.

"My mom always talks about how important it is to be popular, but I'm not sure she really knows what this means to me," Paige, a pretty 14-year-old, told me. "According to her, being liked by boys and girls alike is really important. I think she has this idea that we all hang out together and maybe there might be some kissing but nothing more than that. By middle school, one of the girls in my class was pregnant. When my mom said some negative things about this girl, I said that she was only doing what everyone else is doing and she was just unlucky. That led to a really unpleasant conversation for my mother and me. In the end, my mother didn't ask me whether I was sexually active, which was weird. I was trying to tell her about the difficulties and pressures in my life, but she just didn't want to hear it. All she did was push me away, so now I speak only with my girl and guy friends. I never talk to her about anything going on in my life, and she still has no idea when I started having sex or that I've been smoking weed since I was 13."

On the other hand, there was Violet, who found that her father, a widower, understood a lot more than she expected.

"My dad started talking about sex with me when I was 12. He talked about his experiences as a teenager, which was a big shock to me. He said it wasn't easy for him to talk about it, but he knew what boys were like and he wanted me to know what to watch out for. He said all boys wanted to have sex, and that scared me. By the time I got to high school, I started listening to his advice, though. In high school, I felt much better about having him meet the boys I went out with. I started bringing boys home, and he would talk to them man to man. Some never came back, which made me really mad at him, because I was afraid I would never get asked out again and the word would get out I had a crazy dad. Turns out the real good guys weren't afraid of my dad and kept coming by, and I learned to figure out who was a good guy and who wasn't. One of the guys told me he was glad to meet my dad because he spoke to him about things his parents never spoke to him about. He was referring to sex, protection, and STDs, which my dad came right out and talked about with anyone my age who came by my house.

"I'm sure that even though I still went through the normal teenage drama of 'He loves me...he loves me not' and 'Will he leave me if I don't hook up with him?' I didn't feel as insecure as some of my girlfriends and I didn't feel obligated to go all the way, so I never had to deal with being afraid of getting pregnant or getting STDs. My dad made me feel so good about having him around, I didn't need the guys at school to give me attention, so I didn't have sex before I was ready. When it was time to go to college, my dad told me that he expected me to enjoy myself, but he stressed that the next four years were about studying a lot and preparing for my life as an adult. He kept on telling me that he was proud of me and that I didn't need to have sex or constantly look for male attention to make me feel good about myself. He did such a good job of protecting and reassuring me during high school that I listened to him about college too. In fact, I texted him, at times many times a day, to get his advice and opinion during those years, and it turns out everything he told me helped me become the person I am today. He was right, and his way of talking about everything helped me more than I could have ever expected."

Violet became a lawyer and is married to a supportive and respectful man. She has been weathering life's storms smartly and solidly, and now, with her own children, is continuing the involved and committed parenting her dad modeled for her.

Teenagers in our modern society do have sex. That's one of the many reasons it is so important to provide them with solid support and caring information. They need parents who aren't afraid to tell the truth, no matter how difficult, uncomfortable it may be. In my experience, both in my practice and personally, I watch teens act out and become promiscuous and get seriously into drugs and alcohol when they feel unseen, unvalidated, and unheard. Far too many of my teen patients tell me they resent and even hate their parents. Interestingly, the teens who get into trouble are from both extremes of the economic spectrum, the wealthiest and the poorest. I believe that is because they have to deal with the same things: emotional and physical neglect and lack of supervision. At the wealthy end of the spectrum, absent and often busy and self-involved parents may use money, boarding schools, and household help to substitute for their presence, emotionally and physically. At the poor end, parental involvement is missing often because of financial needs leading parents to work multiple jobs, lack of access to education and, alcohol and drug use.

Melissa was 16 when I started to see her as a patient. She came from a well-to-do East Coast family. Over the course of four years between the ages of 12 and 16, this intellectually curious girl who was brilliant in math was thrown out of three boarding schools and gained more than 50 pounds. She also got into serious trouble with drugs and alcohol. Her family was financially supportive, willing to do anything to help her clean up her act. Unfortunately, a constantly angry Melissa believed her parents had just dumped her into boarding school to get rid of her, and she didn't want anything to do with their help. She became highly promiscuous and a danger to herself and others, dealing drugs and living a highly dangerous life. In desperation, her parents forced Melissa into therapy, and, at the suggestion of the therapist, they sent her to an Outward Bound–type teen rehabilitation program. She was gone for more than three months, during which time she never contacted her family. In fact, after the three months, Melissa asked to stay at the rehab center. She refused to come home. Her parents took a stand and refused to continue paying for the exorbitantly priced program, forcing her to become independent. She chose to work on a farm instead of going home and was gainfully employed as a farm-hand, along with a few friends she'd met in the program who chose the same path.

A year later, Melissa decided to come home, and, while her disdain for her parents hadn't improved much, she remained drug-free and her behavior at school improved remarkably. She asked to get help with her weight and started to act more like the daughter they had been hoping for. Working with me, she began to drop her excess weight and now, at 19, she's excelling in advanced algebra and is much more at peace with her life. Lately, she's even started going to family therapy with her parents. One thing her mother says is that she thinks Melissa learned impulse control during her year away from home. To me this is a great step forward for a girl who was almost lost a mere two years ago.

WHAT'S A PARENT TO DO?

Whether the parental guidance is good or not so great, it's in every teen's job description to separate emotionally from his or her parents in order to become an independent adult. Ideally this happens in such a way that both parent and child develop separate lives but remain close, advancing their relationship to a higher level of communication and mutual respect. The goal is for the young adult and the parent to end up with an interdependent adult relationship. All parents must be prepared for this transition. It is only normal, and even if it does involve dangerous acting out, it is another of life's passages that parents have to deal with in the best possible way. To get through it, they must be present—not just physically, but also emotionally. Parents must learn to listen and validate their teens and set real-life examples by helping the teens find ways to channel their sexuality into positives, helping them become contributors to society and forestall alcohol and drug abuse. It's up to the parents to set clear boundaries to make sure they help their teens and don't abdicate their role as parents and role models. Parents who set good examples for their teens will find that their teens tend to make fewer and less dangerous mistakes as they become healthy, smart, and successful adults. Let's not forget that teens are very fragile as they transition into adulthood. They may put on a tough facade, but don't be fooled. Your teen is very few years away from being the little child who held your hand when you crossed the street. Teens must be acknowledged and reassured as well as listened to carefully. If you want your teen to listen *to you*, make sure *you* listen to your teen.

Sex is part of life, and experimentation is what teens do. It's human nature. So, while we cannot keep them from thinking of sex or hooking up, or even having sex, we can help keep their hormones from getting them into life-demolishing trouble.

Anyone who has come to me and said, "How do I stop my kid from having sex?" hasn't listened to his or her child.

You cannot stop them, but you can help them moderate the need and the actions. You can help them integrate intimacy, connection, and love into their sexuality from the very start.

In my experience, young women are the greatest casualty of our society's obsession with sex. The most effective method of improving outcome is to teach by example. The key to success is to help young women develop solid self-esteem. Teaching women not to equate social popularity with personal success is crucial. While our society urges young women to judge their bodies against impossible and unrealistic ideals, mothers and fathers can teach them to value and accept their bodies as they are. It starts with teaching them to look at themselves in kindness with acceptance, to become familiar with every part of their bodies, to understand how their bodies function—while removing shame and fear from the picture. I spend many highly productive hours with my young women patients, encouraging them to look at their vaginas in the mirror, feel their breasts in the shower, and look at their faces in the mirror without judgment. Young women are so delicate that they can easily break emotionally under the heavy pressures to conform our society places on them. If we teach them to see themselves independently of the outside opinion, they can surely become the strong, self-reliant women every mother hopes her daughter will be.

At the same time, we must teach boys to respect women by modeling a healthy dynamic at home. How boys see their parents behave toward each other is how they will behave as well. If the father treats the mother well and is a true partner, loyal, and a kind best friend, if the parents communicate openly and honestly and are truly connected to each other, the son will respect women and will not be as likely to get involved in rainbow parties, stripper parties, and other activities that lead to the treatment of girls and women as playthings. Sure, every boy experiments, and so does every girl, but if a boy's family atmosphere is one of respect and kindness toward women, he will develop healthy relationships with young women from the very start.

It's a tall order to try to change the present teen paradigm, but we must start someplace, and that is with ourselves. The only option we have for improvement is to lead by example. As adults, we have to be present to provide respectful support and not turn over our teens' lives and sexualities to negative cultural influences. Parents have to stop being afraid of their teens. Experimenting with sex—and drugs—is common, pervasive, and even acceptable in many segments of our society. No matter how many material gifts we give them, or what high-status boarding school or college we pay for, if we leave our children without strong guidance, if they see us behaving poorly, we leave them unprepared for a successful adulthood.

How teenagers cope with their new, hormone-filled bodies within their social and cultural environments may preview how they will define their sexualities through most of their lives. In the rest of this book, we'll see how some of the different scenarios we have seen play out over the course of a lifetime.

CHAPTER 4

WILL YOU LOVE ME TOMORROW?

*"I realized I had just entered an interesting chapter in
my life. I had outgrown the boys of my past and not
quite grown into the men of my future."*

—Carrie Bradshaw, *Sex and the City*

"I remember that moment," my patient Jessica said to me. "That
first moment when I closed the door to my very own apartment,
poured myself a glass of wine from my own refrigerator, and
kicked off my shoes after my first day at my first real job. The
feeling was exhilarating. I was finally an adult, an independent
woman. Life stretched out ahead of me, and I was going to have
it all—a powerful career, an amazing relationship, and definitely
someday a family. I never could have foreseen then that the
search for the right guy would take me into my 40s."

When you're in your 20s, the season of sex feels like a
steamy, endless summer. You can't imagine a future that doesn't
go on forever. You think your choices are unlimited and your

body will be forever young, sexy, and dynamic. In fact, you don't even think. You just can't wait to get on with your life. Maybe you've graduated from college and moved out of your parents' home, maybe you share living space with your girlfriends, or, like Jessica, even manage to have your own apartment. You are an adult, no longer accountable to parental rules or supervision. Some young adults in the present economic climate are forced to become "boomerang kids" and temporarily move back in with their parents, but even in those arrangements, the parent-child dynamic has changed. From here on it has to be understood that the decisions you make and the actions you take have consequences that you alone are responsible for. You can no longer blame your parents for bad outcomes or get grounded to keep you out of trouble. You are now on your own, for real.

That includes the choices you make about sex.

For many young men and women, the years immediately following high school and college fall along the spectrum of yet another decade of experimentation. This often takes the form of uncommitted and carefree sex and risk-taking that are perceived by our society as inconsequential, yet another rite of passage. You're sowing your wild oats—it's all just part of being young. This is the time when, many young men and women find themselves partying till dawn and having sex with a number of often nameless and unmemorable partners. One-night stands are certainly a rite of passage at this time in most people's lives.

I had a pretty young female receptionist once who was smart and efficient. She was right out of an upstate junior college and brand new to all the temptations New York City had to offer.

Within a few months of starting in my office she changed. With increasing frequency, she came to work wearing the same clothes she had worn the day before. Overtired and unfocused on her performance, texting all day, whispering on the phone about her one-night stands and perpetual hangovers, she was following the examples of her media role models. She was doing exactly what she thought she ought to do. Our society accepts and even condones this type of behavior as the norm for young women.

After a few weeks of watching her lose interest in her job due to exhaustion from her extracurricular activities, I talked to her. I told her that her social life was negatively affecting her performance and keeping her from doing a good job. Enjoying the perceived freedom of being young and single is one thing—but letting it diminish your potential and interfering with your productivity is another. Free of parental rules, she felt she needed to just let her hair down. I told her she was jeopardizing her future and she would do better if she consciously tried to balance her social and work life better. Fortunately, she heard my comments and started limiting her partying to weekends. Her performance at work greatly improved, and both she and the work environment benefitted. Today, she runs a large section of an office with more than 20 employees, and she's only 30 years old.

Young adults in their 20s believe they are immortal. To them, daring and often reckless activities like extreme sports, drug and alcohol abuse, and spur-of-the-moment sex fall into the category of *carpe diem* (seize the day). They often believe that risky business enriches the tapestry of their lives, expands their horizons, and gives them wisdom, but they rarely consider the possibility that dangerous behavior could lead to disaster instead.

While our American culture is rooted deeply in the Puritan morals of our forefathers and foremothers, it's the new world opened up by the 1960s and its sexual revolution that fuel the behavior that most of today's 20-somethings emulate. The image of alluring free hookups with no strings attached dominates the popular media. In romantic comedies and dramas on the screen, on book covers, in the pages of popular magazines, and on the internet, including social media, youth is equated with hard, young bodies; freedom from commitment; and abundant, easy, crazy, wild sex.

But all too often there is a huge contradiction here that may lead to problems: While romanticizing casual sex, young people are also concomitantly given the message that they're supposed to start looking for a lifetime mate. How do young men and women find a serious, committed relationship while they're trying to live up to the messages of casual, exciting, and unimportant sex? The confusion is created and reinforced by the unreasonable expectations from a culture that confuses fairy tales with real love and intimacy—and then ties them all to sex.

For young women, this contradiction is particularly stressful and confusing. There is a long, winding, pothole-filled road on the way to finding "the right one."

The sexual revolution has opened the door for women to compete with men in the professional world and prove they can be just as successful and accomplished in erstwhile male-dominated careers. Just look at what happened to medicine and law, two male-dominated professions only 20 years ago.

More than 40 years ago, when I applied to medical school, I was one of very few women attempting to enter the profession. Medicine was solidly and unshakably a boys' club. During my application process, some of the male physicians who interviewed me asked questions like, "Why should we take you into medical school over a man?" Or they'd make barbed comments like, "You will certainly get pregnant and waste a very expensive education" and, "Accepting a woman into medical school is a waste of time, because most drop out to have children and stay home." Who would ever believe these attitudes were totally acceptable as recently as the 1970s? Being perceived as a sex object and not as an intellectual equal was the rule, not the exception.

As the women's liberation movement helped us start to equalize the playing field, it also opened the door for the sexual revolution. There's one problem—the sexual revolution never took into account that in terms of physical and sexual needs and desires, men and women are quite different. I've practiced medicine now for more than 35 years, and, while much has changed to help us move toward equality for women, the trade-offs have often been very harsh and the price way too high, with many unexpected and unaddressed outcomes that are still difficult to integrate for both sexes. I can tell you that few of my female patients—myself included—have ever lived the carefree *Sex and the City* fantasy without some serious bruises and disappointments. In my experience, casual sex is still too often a setup for emotional trauma for too many women. Remember, not all men were raised in households hailing women as equals. There are still too many boys raised to have very little respect for women. And no matter what we say, these boys become men who have no respect for women and cause significant damage to relationships and the women involved in them. Much of the trouble starts when young women unknowingly fall for "the bad boy."

THE WRONG KIND OF MAN

Regardless of geography or socioeconomic condition, young women in college, in their early to mid-20s, too often hold on to the image of the popular high school or college jock as the definition of the most desirable mate. Is the handsome bad boy who parties all night and goes through women like popcorn really the best choice when a woman is in search of a real partner? For some women, the answer is yes, and biology might hold a potential answer.

According to a study published in September 2013 in the *Proceedings of the National Academy of Sciences of the United States of America*, men with smaller testicles might be more likely to be more nurturing fathers than men with larger testicles.[1]

According to the *Harvard Gazette* marriage drops testosterone in men[2] and once children arrive in the marriage, men whose testosterone levels drop are more likely to be directly involved in child-rearing than those whose testosterone levels stay high.[3]

Lots of factors affect testosterone levels and size of testicles, and all are tied into a man's nurturing abilities. A book by biological anthropologist Robert Martin, titled *How We*

Do It: The Evolution and Future of Human Reproduction (Basic Books, 2013), raises the possibility that "a man can either invest in looking after the child of one wife, or he can invest more in sperm production if he has several wives."

Anthropology, biology, and social science all converge in their attempt to figure out what the ingredients are that we should be looking for when we decide to pair off. We already know that environmental influences change biology.

But the question looming ever larger at this time in women's lives is, what type of man should women look for to be a partner?

So many of my patients tell me story after story about wrong choices in men. Regardless of the size of men's testicles or testosterone levels, there is a multitude of difficult and clearly wrong types of guys to hook up with if you honestly are looking for a good mate and a solid father for your kids. Unfortunately, in our society the wrong guys are all too often 20- to 30-year-old good-looking, competitive, successful, funny, athletic, well-dressed, and confident men—the heartthrobs of many insecure women with low self-esteem who are sadly misdirected.

Sasha, a beautiful 28-year-old Russian-trained biochemist, came to the U.S. and promptly met John, a highly successful 35-year-old bond trader. He was very attractive both physically and socially. John knew everyone in town and had lots of college and high school friends and a full social calendar. Sasha was impressed, and within three months she proudly told me that she was now his "arm candy and loving it." He professed his love for her, showered her with expensive gifts, and told her he would even bring her family over from Moscow. Their sex life was full of passion and excitement, and they never had their fill of each other. They had sex at least two or three times every day. Sasha believed John was her knight in shining armor and started making plans to move in with him.

About a week before the move was planned, something happened. John stopped calling her the usual 10 times a day, and his texts became sporadic and brief. She assumed he was busy with work. The day before the big move, Sasha received a call from a woman who told her that she too had been dating John at the same time. As the two women got into a real conversation, it became clear they were pretty much at the same point in their poorly perceived relationship with John. He had made similar declarations of love and commitment to the other woman too. Sasha was stunned and devastated. She did not want to believe the woman but had a gut feeling she was telling the truth. She thought about how some women are competitive and out to hurt each other. However, in this case, Sasha felt it important to heed the woman's story. That evening, Sasha asked John to have dinner with her to set up the moving details. He met her and acted as if everything were normal. While he went to the bathroom she went through his cell phone. Sasha found texts from at least 10 women she knew from their social circle, and was shocked. His texts to and from them were all filled with sexual innuendo and details she would have preferred not to read—clearly, he was sleeping with all of them! Crushed, Sasha ran out of the restaurant before John came back from the men's room.

Guys like John are often referred to as the type who needs to sow his seed but in the process is just a bad guy who treats women badly and leaves behind a trail of distraught and disappointed women. These guys have a facade that's irresistible, but their inability to commit and deliver on a long-term intimate relationship reveals a side of men women must carefully protect themselves from or pay long-lasting and very high emotional consequences.

When they do finally settle down with one woman for a while, these "bad boys" don't usually change. Somehow, they seem to choose women who won't ask much of them emotionally and who are just thrilled to be chosen as "the one." These women become their doormats, while the men continue their busy lives as matadors. When these popular males do settle down, it's often temporary. They are the most likely to be among the 50 percent of Americans who cheat on their partners.[4] As age takes its toll, and as time and society turn the popular guys every woman wants into family men with ever-expanding responsibilities and waistlines, too many of them still refuse to change—they continue their duplicitous behavior no matter the cost. Many eventually get divorced, and some have multiple marriages full of drama, bitter child custody battles, and child-support and alimony fights following them throughout their unsettled and often uncaring, poorly prioritized lives.

On the other hand, according to the small-testicle theory, the quiet, less attractive guy—the shy "geek" who spends his high school years unnoticed by the popular girls—may be more likely to be a solid and intimate partner. Less likely to be a womanizer and more likely to settle down with one woman, this type of man is mostly monogamous and a reliable partner, provider, and highly involved parent. This is the type of man who understands intimacy and combines it with sexuality, achieving a healthy and responsible marriage.

I remember in my 20s, I thought I'd never get old. No young people think they will get old or die. It's a fact of life. Unfortunately, this fantasy of eternal youth and immortality prevents many 20-something women from thinking ahead and rationally evaluating the long-term consequences of many of the choices they make. This includes what type of man they seek to partner with for the long run.

My patient Jo is a smart, highly educated 30-year-old writer who spent her college years being the life of the party. During her senior year she met Marcus, a professor of English literature, with whom she fell madly in love. He was 20 years her senior and on his third marriage when they met. He told her he loved children and had them in each marriage. At school, he had a reputation for being a ladies' man, but that did not deter Jo, who was sure she was the one with whom he would settle down permanently. She believed she would be able to tame this tiger. The passionate love affair they started was a whirlwind of heady sex, alcohol, and marijuana.

It took a short few months for Marcus to separate from his wife so he could devote every possible moment to the new love of his life. While waiting for his third divorce to come through, he took Jo on trips around the world, where he would lecture while she sat in the audience, riveted to his every word. They made love many times every day, everywhere, with gusto and excitement. To Jo, sex was an expression of their love, connection, deep intimacy, and intellectual compatibility. Shortly after his separation, they moved in together and life continued in a fog of passion and sex for almost five years. One day, as their life together started to settle into a routine, Jo realized she was ready to have children of her own and, for the first time, raised the subject of marriage. Nonplussed, Marcus told her he was done with children and had no intention of ever marrying again. He told her he loved her but that the freedom and excitement of their no-strings-attached relationship made her highly desirable to him. He didn't want to change that arrangement.

Jo couldn't hear him: Her biology was calling, and she wanted to take their relationship to the next level. Instead of reaching a compromise or opening a deeper discussion and seeking professional help, they ended the conversation without a plan. As a result, a chasm opened between them. Marcus stopped taking Jo to conferences, and within six months their passionate love affair just died. One night Marcus came home and sullenly announced that he was moving out. Jo learned he had met a new woman at a conference and, as with Jo years before, had decided that *this* time it was *real* love, for sure. Jo swore off men, and, after almost a year of being depressed, started dating again. She spent a few years fluctuating between dating men and women, and finally fell in love with a woman whom she eventually married, had two children with, and built a happy life with.

> ### LOW SEX DRIVE CAN START EARLY
>
> If you are in your 20s and not married, there are other factors besides hormones and cultural mores that are impacting your sex drive. In the National Health and Social Life Survey (NHSLS)[5], conducted through the University of Chicago, women in their 20s who weren't married felt more anxiety about their sexual performance than married women did. Additionally, the single women experienced more difficulty climaxing. As far as desire for sex was concerned, it was linked to frequency. The less often the women had sex, the less they wanted it.

SEX AND THE CITY IS FICTION, NOT A HANDBOOK!

Most women in their 20s and early 30s are determined to find the perfect mate. They also expect and accept that, along the way, they will have to kiss a lot of frogs. That's probably an understatement for the variety and types of sexual experiences today's women go through in the quest for the "right" guy.

Many patients who come to me right out of college don't think twice before hopping into bed for a one-night stand, a.k.a. hook-up that means nothing more than "just fun" to either party.

Kate, at 23, is one such example.

"The day I moved into my own bedroom in the apartment I shared with three other women, I was happy as a clam," the vibrant redhead told me. "I could do what I wanted, and I knew it was party time. In college, I didn't date a lot, so I was ready to have some fun. I'd go out with a group of girlfriends to the local bars, where there was never a shortage of guys. The goal is to meet a guy and hook up for the night and make sure no one makes a big deal out of it. If I'm attracted to someone, and he to me, we'll have sex and sometimes spend the night together. I always hope he calls again the next day, but if he doesn't, I've learned from all my other girl and guy friends, it's not a big deal. My generation doesn't 'date' the way my parents did. We don't need to waste time being wined and dined to have sex. We'd rather hang out with friends and just hook up when the mood strikes. Sure, I want to get married someday, but I want to live a little—no, make that a lot—before I settle down with one guy for the rest of my life. I'm young and this is my time to enjoy it. I come from the generation after *Sex and the City*, and we are even freer and clearer about sex than Carrie Bradshaw and her friends were. How will I know what I'm really looking for if I don't play around with a lot of guys now when I'm young and free? My parents were divorced when I was 12, and I watched both of them go crazy with dating and lots of sex partners when they were middle-aged. I don't want to be like them. I want to live a wild and crazy life now, figure out what I am looking for in a man, and then settle down with the right guy for me so I'll never get divorced."

Kate's view of marriage was clearly shaped by her family's example. It sounds as if she believes married life might be a sexual death sentence leading to divorce, with the 20s being like the last meal before the execution. Kate is a great example of how upbringing plays a very strong role in the way sex and marriage are perceived. When kids see their parents desperately unhappy in their marriages, or see them getting divorced and becoming highly sexual afterward to make up for years of sexual deprivation, young women will often take an opposite path. What better way to express their rebellion against the parents' lifestyles than through unbridled sexuality as early in life as possible?

But while so many young people live sexually and emotionally uncommitted lives, they persist in the magical thinking that a committed and permanent relationship will miraculously appear for them when the time is right. Most of the 20-something young women I meet first tell me they are perfectly comfortable with a life of casual sex, but when I start to probe deeper, they admit they're confused by the mixed messages they're getting from society. Who wouldn't be, when the implication is, "Go ahead and have sex with anyone, while at the same time, search for the man you want a real relationship with that should last a lifetime." Too many young women are indoctrinated into believing that casual sex makes them equal to men. This idea is confusing and demeaning. At 29, my patient Trish is a perfect example of this conflict.

"I'm really confused," she told me. "I definitely want to find a great guy and settle down soon, but the closer I get to 30, the more I fear that finding the right guy isn't likely to happen. I am getting frantic and I know it. All my girlfriends are either settling down or also running scared. For years, I've been having sex with guys, and I just assumed that having fun sex will eventually lead to a real connection when I meet the right guy for me. I feel like Kristen Wiig's character in *Bridesmaids*—falling into tons of sexual hook-ups with guys, hoping that if I'm sexy enough and always ready for booty calls, one of them will eventually want a serious relationship with me. Oddly, that hasn't happened yet. I feel like I'm on a treadmill of dead-end hook-ups and I'm running out of time. So I ask friends and family to set me up with guys who might be right, but once I meet someone I like, I honestly have no clue how to handle it. I don't know whether to sleep with the guy first or try to become friends. Some of my girlfriends say wait three dates, others tell me they found their husband in a bar and slept with him the first night they met. It's a lot of stress and no one has the answer. The lucky ones just find the right guy, while people like me just keep searching and hoping the next one will be it."

When I asked Trish if she ever considered the male point of view, she told me, "Of course I do. My girlfriends and I talk about it all the time. We all agree men just want sex. When we were kids, my mom always told my sister and me that all boys ever want is to get into your pants. My mom also told us never to have sex on a first date, because then the guy will lose respect for us. She's so old-fashioned; I believe her advice doesn't apply to us, so I can't even listen to her blabber. She's just annoying, and what does she know about being my age anyway? But I know she's right even though I would never admit it to her. Men want sex, and if you don't give it to them, it's just so easy for them to get it elsewhere. They don't wait, like in her youth; they just move on. They never run out of women willing to sleep with them. I'm not sure I know what makes a guy stay with one particular woman. It seems like a crapshoot to me and most of my friends. There are so many women willing to have sex and just do anything to be with a guy; it's scary out there. The competition is so fierce, and women are so catty and awful to one another. They just want to get their hands on the guy and don't care how they do it or how they hurt others in the process. It's really hard to be in your 20s in my generation."

When I ask young men like Ralph, 32, what their perspective is, the answer is quite simple and to the point. "There are so many women around, and they are all available to have sex with; there's no shortage of easy hook-ups. I don't have a biological clock and have no good reason to worry about getting married or having kids. I'm happy with work, my life, and my buddies, and we all agree that it's the women who want to get married and have kids. We could just go through life like this forever. We don't have any pressing reason to change. It's the women who push us, and if we fall in love or get pushed hard enough by a woman we may think we love, or sex is so great with her we can't stop wanting her, we just go along and get married. And sometimes we regret it, because the women really want to get married to have kids, and they change the moment you put a ring on their finger, and we the guys are left with these obsessed women who want family and kids while we don't really care much about it. I don't want to speak for other guys, but I know my friends and I would rather have our time together to play and travel and watch sports and enjoy each other's company and be left alone by these all-too-often-crazy women. Sometimes I think the price for having sex with only one woman gets to be too high, and unless we hold on to our life very hard, they just change everything for us."

There you go. An honest man telling a terribly hard truth for women to hear.

Like young men, young women in their prime have hormones that make them want sex, so why shouldn't they just have sex? Women like Trish in search of meaningful relationships in a sea of casual sex and lots of deceptive people are at a terrible disadvantage. Trish can have sex with her date right away and then hope he'll call again and want to get to know her better. But if all his dates approach the situation in the same casual fashion, what reason does he have to slow down and form a bond with any of them? How does he even notice her as different from all the other women throwing themselves at him? If Trish holds out, delaying or refusing sex in order to develop a less superficial connection with a man and make herself noticed by him, she lives in fear she'll lose him to another woman who won't make him wait. But then, why would any woman want to be with a man she has to convince to stay with her? If a woman has self-esteem and knows her worth, she will not allow herself to be a player in the world that devalues women and places them in untenable positions.

If men and women become honest and start talking to each other about how they really feel, then maybe the transition from random sex to meaningful, loving, intimate, and committed sex will become smoother and more equal for both. If men and women can get on the same page sexually and emotionally, things may get easier, and fewer disappointments may define their lives. Less game-playing and more honesty lead to more mutual respect and long-term, intimate, and kind relationships. It doesn't matter what the tabloids tell you.

Trish referred to another quote from *Sex and the City*—which, while an entertaining TV series, is too often interpreted by young women as the ideal and most desirable how-to relationship manual for strong, emancipated, and modern single young women. A character from the show laments, "Men are like taxicabs. When they're ready to get married, they turn their light on. The next woman they pick up, boom! They marry." Trish agrees. "With men, it's all about timing. When the guy is ready, whichever woman walks through the door next is the right one. It's not the same with women. We're not only forced to figure out who's the right guy, we also have to get in there at exactly the right moment—for *him*! It's not fair. The decks are just totally stacked against us." Given Ralph's comments, Trish may very well be totally right. I listen to young women every day, and the ones who understand and integrate the importance of self-esteem and confidence do well and live fulfilling lives, while those who try to emulate what people like the characters *in Sex and the City* say or do usually wind up sad and disappointed in relationships created by checklists instead of true love and intimacy.

There's even more to consider. From what some of my male patients tell me, maybe the men she hooks up with think that she'll have sex with anyone and don't trust her to be loyal in the long term. Perhaps some of them really want to connect but feel Trish is probably just out for a good time and that *she's* the one using *them*. Harvard urologist Abraham Morgentaler, MD, has written a book called *Why Men Fake It: The Totally Unexpected Truth about Men and Sex*, which brings to light the deeply conflicted feelings many men have in our age of sexual freedom, when so many men and women jump into bed just for sex without intimacy or any consideration for possible consequences. Morgentaler's research shows that men are just as confused and even scared and embarrassed about the ever-diminishing amount of intimacy and connection in their sex lives, trying to please women and hitting the cultural roadblocks often as frequently as the women. Maybe the problem doesn't lie just with the men. Maybe women need to look at themselves without the outside influences and figure out who they are and what they honestly want in their personal lives.

My patient Laura worries about all of this. Her story is different from Kate's and Trish's, but it's one I hear from many patients in her age group.

"John and I met the first week in college, and we've been together ever since," she told me. "Our families got close and even celebrate holidays together now. We moved in together once we graduated and never looked at ourselves as separate from each other. We do everything together. It's now seven years since we moved into our own place, and John is dragging his feet about asking me to marry him. I know it's not a money issue, because we both work and make a good living. Sometimes we even talk about getting engaged; he says we should do it, but then somehow it never happens. It's like he's just stuck. I always wanted to be a young mom, to have my kids when I was in my 20s and early 30s. But the longer this goes on, the more my vision for my life gets pushed back. We have more fights about getting married than about anything else. Almost every day something triggers me, and I'll ask when he's planning to propose. He pushes back and says, 'I don't understand what the problem is. We are living together and are committed to each other. Why are you in such a rush?'

"What he says sort of makes sense, but then I remember all the stuff I watch on TV and on Facebook and I start to wonder if we *are* truly committed to each other. I know about this girl who lived with her boyfriend for 10 years, and then one day he just walked out and she never saw him again. There is so much out there about terrible things that happen; I want to hold on to John and just get married, and then I'll feel totally safe. If he loves me so much and wants to spend his life with me, then what's stopping him from moving on to the next phase? Why doesn't he just give me a ring and plan a wedding with me? To be perfectly honest, the longer these stupid arguments go on, the more insecure I get and the less I'm attracted to him sexually. We used to have such great sex; I know it was one of the reasons we got together to begin with. With every passing week with all the stupid arguments and stress, I watch myself losing interest in him. Wanting him sexually should have nothing to do with whether we are engaged or not, but somehow, I am watching our sex life just wither away, and I have no idea why. Recently I started thinking of leaving him. I even put a time limit on the whole thing in my mind. I said if he doesn't give me an engagement ring by my birthday, I'm out of this relationship. I don't have time to waste anymore. Then I'll think, "But John is such a great guy. How can I leave after seven years and start over with someone else? Why is this ring-and-marriage thing so important anyway?"

Every Thursday, Laura and her girlfriends from college and high school go out to a local diner to eat, drink, and talk. When she talks to them about her doubts and fears about her relationship with John, she doesn't get enough help or insight. Her girlfriends who are still out looking for a mate tell her she should count her blessings that she's found a good man. They tell her horror stories of disastrous affairs and horrific relationships with cheating and lying womanizers or alcoholics, gamblers, or drug addicts, who cover up the truth for years—and when the truth comes out, it's too late for the women to make a change that is not devastating. Some of Laura's friends do advise her to keep waiting for John to decide when the time is right; they are sure he will propose eventually and everything will work out. She calls them the blind optimists. Others tell her to just leave him and move on, because she certainly has given him enough time and if he can't hear her and do what she wants now, how is he going to behave in 10 years' time when there are kids around? Better to cut her losses and move on. Laura is confused and scared. She has invested so much time and effort, she has no idea what to do. The frustration is affecting her work and making her feel less sexual and more desperate. When she asks her mom for advice, she gets no help at all. Her mom has been with her dad for more than 30 years and says, "All men are alike. Unless it's their idea, they don't budge." She tells Laura to stop whining and just wait.

"Is this what the 20s are supposed to be like?" Laura says. "It's all drama, and I feel like it's all made up by someone else's expectations for my life. What is my life anyway?" Laura always thought her 20s were supposed to be the most exciting time of her life, not a tug of war. She's not alone in this sea of confusion, fear, and loss of personal identity.

INTIMACY AND SEXUALITY

When young women talk to me about their sex lives, they always use the words "intimacy" and "love." In spite of the casual attitude perpetuated by the idea of hook-ups among the young and carefree, being intimate—even in a young woman's world— is often synonymous with sex. This puzzles me. When I look up "intimacy" in the dictionary, I don't see "sex" on the list of synonyms. "Intimacy" is defined as emotional closeness—a quality my young patients tell me is pretty much lacking in most of their dealings with young men that involve sex. When a relationship lacks emotional closeness, how can it ever be meaningful, deep, and long-lasting? Many of the 20-something-year-old patients I see are caught in a trap set by our society: They define their self-worth by how sexually desirable they are, yet they long for a man who will appreciate them as individuals, real women. They long for closeness, trust, and connection, but when they try to find these things through instant sex based on chemical attraction alone, they hit a wall. They are searching for love and instead get casual sex.

On functional MRIs the brain regions that are activated during orgasm include sensory, motor, reward, frontal cortical, and brainstem regions, areas of the brain also activated when women experience connection. All this can easily be extrapolated to feelings of love and care.[6]

Delicate, short-haired, and stylishly dressed Jan, age 26, described a nightmare story all too common among women in her age group.

"Michael and I met at a party and hooked up," she told me. "He was smart and funny and spent the entire evening flirting with me and making me laugh. We sat on the floor and drank tequila and talked for hours. By the end of the party we were both really hammered, and I invited him up to my apartment. We had sex that night, and it was great even though I don't remember much about the details. A few days later he finally called me. I had been watching my phone every five minutes waiting for his call the entire time. He asked me to come over, and I went to his place and we had a few drinks, smoked a joint, and had sex again. It was really great. A few days later, it was back to my apartment. In hindsight, it quickly became a once-or twice-a-week booty call. I was bummed that we never went to dinner or the movies; we never went out with his or my friends. We only met for sex, but I didn't want to scare him away by being too pushy about going out, so I didn't say a thing. I figured in time he would come around and see how nice I was, and he would figure out it was time to have a real relationship.

"Then one day he texted me at work and asked me if I wanted to go on a ski weekend with him and his buddies. I was so excited—I was sure this was a sign he liked me and we were moving in the right direction, so I immediately agreed to go. I've never been on skis and hate ice and snow, but I really liked the guy and after all, we were finally leaving the bedroom. Immediately, my fantasy took over. I pictured us becoming a real couple, going après-ski to the lodge with his friends, then sleeping in the lodge in a bedroom with a big four-poster bed, cuddling together under down comforters, watching the snow fall and sharing intimate secrets and having great sex. I had no doubt this was going to be a fantastic weekend that would bring us closer and move our budding relationship along. Unfortunately, it didn't turn out that way.

"The first day at the resort, Michael put on his ski gear, pointed me to the beginner's trail, and headed off toward the black diamond slope with his friends. Several hours—and falls—later, cold and tired, I went looking for him. I found him at the bar, where he was already partying with a large group of people. Happy to be indoors, I didn't even think it weird he hadn't looked for me on the slopes. Even more strangely, he just waved a quick hello when I arrived, focused on talking to his buddies and barely noticing me. So I joined him and his friends for dinner and more drinks. I really felt left out as they all joked and talked about people I'd never met and things and places I knew nothing about. It wasn't that bad, but I wished he had treated me better. Finally, late at night, the party ended and we went back to our room. Instead of the romantic evening I'd been dreaming of, Michael just passed out on the bed. This was pretty much the story for the four very long days and even longer nights we spent on our so-called together ski vacation. By the time it was over, I was an emotional wreck. My mind kept playing tricks on me. On one hand, I felt rejected and alone; on the other, I was hoping things would improve if only I was sweeter and kept a smile on my face longer and looked better and acted like everything was just fine. I texted my friends asking for opinions, and some said I was doing the right thing while others told me to get on the first train and come back home and dump the SOB. Of course, I stayed.

"It wasn't until the drive back that I got the courage to ask him why he wanted me to come at all if he planned to just ignore me the whole time. Without making eye contact, Michael told me, 'I knew that every one of my friends was bringing a date. I didn't want to show up alone, and I thought you would like it.' I was so disappointed. Looking back, I don't think Michael was a bad guy. I guess we never really knew each other, since our entire relationship was limited to just having sex. I should never have gone with him, or at least I could've talked to him about my expectations the first time he left me alone on the slopes. Instead, I kept quiet and miserable because I didn't want to rock the boat. What is wrong with me? Why did I sell myself so short, for a guy I didn't even know? Why am I so desperate to just be with a guy? Any guy."

With women's struggle for sexual freedom and gender equality, have we created problems we never anticipated? Why do so many young women allow themselves to be treated badly just to be able to say they are part of a couple? Why are so many young women afraid to tell men the truth about how they feel and think? Why do young women fear being alone so much that they allow themselves to be abused just to be part of a couple? Why are so many young women regressing when it comes to equality in sex and intimate relationships? It's heartbreaking to see young women's stories played out over and over again as if 50 years of struggle for women's equality never existed or has made little impact. Why encourage men to treat women badly instead of showing them the beauty and kindness of women as an example to follow?

THE RIGHT ONE

While party girls enjoy their youth by following the examples of the drama-filled lives of reality TV celebrities and keep struggling with difficult times brought on by unkind, commitment-phobic men with infinite numbers of young women ready to jump into bed with them, there are still plenty of women who are looking to get married and start a family in their 20s. These women are not following the trends; they're following in their parents' cultural footsteps and religious and cultural mores, sometimes having to go all-out against the tide. These are the women who are aware of their biological clock and the pressure to get married and have children. Whether or not these women are pursuing a career at the same time, the search for an appropriate mate becomes the priority by mid- to late 20s in most women's lives. For men, the imperative to marry and have children isn't even on the horizon. The majority of men at this stage are perfectly happy to party and jump around with multiple sex partners, and only when a woman they fall in love with focuses them on marriage do they follow.

So how is a woman to find the right guy in this fog of sex, drugs, and drinking?

From what I've seen, researched, and listened to, many women meet their future husbands at work or through friends. Others look for compatible guys through activities like sports or music, or through arts or religious groups. And then there's internet dating—now a multibillion-dollar industry. In a very short 20 years, looking for love online has gone from being an embarrassing stigma to being a socially acceptable and often most desirable way to weed out frogs in the search for the prince.

Michelle, 23 years old and with a conservative, religious upbringing, is a modern woman who nevertheless wanted to follow her family tradition when it came to finding "the one." Under the watchful eye of her mother and aunt—both widows in their 40s—Michelle joined Tinder, Match, and eHarmony. The three women would meet on Fridays to decide which guy Michelle should go out with that week. One Friday, they all agreed on George, a young man from their neighborhood who was also a member of their church, although Michelle had never met him. Her mother and aunt knew his family and were quite happy that the two decided to go out. Within a few dates,

Michelle and George were pretty sure the relationship was "it." They had common interests and common backgrounds. Neither was interested in partying or sowing wild oats. They were happy to watch TV after work and go out on weekends to Bible study and church group activities. Their lives fit hand in glove, and they were happy and content. Within a year, they were engaged. Everyone in the family was thrilled as Michelle's life followed her master plan.

George turned out to be a kind, hard-working engineer who shared Michelle's goals of a solid family life. His family became close to Michelle's, and his recently widowed uncle actually started dating Michelle's aunt. Miraculously, that match also led to marriage, and Michelle's family doubled in size and happiness.

While stories like George and Michelle's are extremely common, we don't hear about them a lot. Maybe it is because there is no drama attached to them, or maybe they seem too simple and, some may think, boring. I do hear these stories frequently from my patients who aren't afraid of not fitting into the modern, "cool" world. These people easily manage to find a partner with shared beliefs and also consistently have the support of their families, friends, and cultural institutions. These are people who don't look for fireworks, crazy passion, and large doses of drama but rather focus on creating a life with companions who have similar values and life goals. While many still do their share of partying during the school years, once they are out in the real world, they seem to have a clear life plan and find the right partner to implement that plan with. Passion and good sex are part of many of these relationships, but love, intimacy, commitment, and family values are the driving forces ruling these people's lives.

ARRANGED MARRIAGES?

Arranged marriages are an extreme example of this goal-oriented mating. Though in the U.S. we think of arranged marriages as primitive, even uncivilized, and an insult to our never-ending struggle to achieve total independence from our families, according to some counts, 55 percent or more of all marriages in the world are made by parents or other family members.[7] In the U.S., the divorce rate for first marriages is between 40 and 50 percent,[8] while arranged marriages have less than a 5 percent divorce rate worldwide. That's quite an impressive statistic. While I'm not advocating for modern women and men to switch over to the arranged-marriage system, I think it is very useful to look at how other cultures view marriage, as well as the outcomes in those cultures. There are some important lessons to be learned by examining other systems that regard marriage as a permanent state, rather than as a "maybe" situation with the possibility to get out as soon as things don't work out perfectly.

Let's take the example of my patient Kumar, a handsome and very accomplished second-generation Indian man. Kumar's parents, who emigrated from India three decades ago, watched their Indian-American son follow the "Western way" of courtship for several years, repeatedly choosing women who either broke his heart or did not share his values or life philosophy.

Finally, Kumar's dad stepped in and suggested the centuries-old method of an arranged marriage. Kumar initially rejected the idea. He was American-born and lived a modern life. However, in time he evaluated his dating situation and found it unsatisfying, and decided to go along with his parents' suggestion.

The entire family flew back to India, to the town they had originally come from, and his parents and other relatives got together and interviewed more than 10 young women and their parents. Kumar was out with friends, not involved in the process. The parents chose the quiet, serious Prabal, who was introduced to Kumar the day before their scheduled wedding. Kumar wasn't sure he was doing the right thing, but he knew that looking for a wife in New York for three years had led to nothing but disappointment. He also knew from being an American that things could be undone, should he find the arranged marriage not working for him. He respected and trusted his parents, and had internalized some of their values more than he knew, but he left the door open to just change his mind and go back to American-style dating, just in case. With a lot of hope and mixed emotions, he went ahead with the arranged marriage.

The marriage of Kumar and Prabal got off to a rocky start. Prabal was a shy virgin who came from a world very different from Kumar's. Sex was difficult, and the two clearly didn't have the same degree of experience or expectations in this area. Kumar had had sex with many women during his dating days, while Prabal had never even thought of sex before marriage. Their first few attempts at intercourse left her in tears and him wishing he hadn't listened to his parents. After six weeks in India, a frustrated Kumar went back to the U.S., ready to call the whole thing off. He told me he wasn't sure if he should stick with the marriage. "How am I supposed to love a woman I don't know and I can't even have sex with?" he asked me.

I pointed out that around here, we Americans often marry people we don't know very well either. We just have sex with them first, which only serves to confuse us and give us the false belief that we know each other. Few marriages are like the movie *When Harry Met Sally*, starting out with long-term friendships. And even in those cases, there are no guarantees for success. It's all about giving the relationship time and learning who the other person is while he or she learns who you are. It's about becoming friends and accepting each other as we are. Sex is part of the process, but it isn't *the* process.

Kumar agreed to give the marriage another shot. Prabal bit the bullet and moved to the States. She became Americanized faster than her husband expected. Time flew by and life just happened. They did have sex, and Prabal got pregnant very quickly. They had two sons. Prabal took all her teacher exams and got a job in a school teaching young children, which she had always dreamt of doing. While the first five years were difficult for both, they hung in there and in the process learned how to be partners and parents. Now, 10 years later, they've built one of the strongest marriages I've ever seen. Their family is thriving, Kumar tells me sex is great, and they really love and respect each other. Most importantly, Kumar tells me how much he likes Prabal, and how they are best friends and prefer each other's company to anyone else's.

Does this one example mean arranged marriages are necessarily better? Absolutely not! It's important to remember that despite the low divorce rates for arranged marriages, they come with problems too. In many cultures where arranged marriages are the norm, women are overtly and sadly lower than second-class citizens. In many of these arranged marriages, abuse and oppression of women go hand in hand with severe limitations of women's life choices. I unequivocally denounce those types of marriages. But I do believe that studying arranged marriages (especially the likes of Prabal and Kumar's) sheds light on the fact that often older, more experienced and wise members of the family being part of the decision-making process may be more helpful in making good choices than our youth-focused culture would have us believe. Marriage should be serious business, and getting as much help as possible should be the norm. The same parents whom we thought of as idiots when we were teens may be quite useful when it comes to input on choices for life partners when we are in our 20s and 30s. Having multiple generations together interacting and learning from each other may be one of the best tools for success when it comes to good choices in life partners.

THE DIVORCE EFFECT

One explanation for young men's and women's current sexual behavior might be found in the statistics on divorce from the 1950s to the early 2000s. During that time, the divorce rates in the United States rose dramatically. Many children watched their parents get divorced, sometimes more than once.

In 1950, the divorce rate in the U.S. was 26 percent. Today's baby boomers are statistically likely to have grown up in intact, traditional families. That rate stayed about the same until 17 years later. It wasn't until after 1967, the no-fault divorce laws, and the advent of the full-on sexual revolution that rates shot up exponentially. By 1985 the American divorce rate had reached an estimated 50 percent.

Ironically, it's likely that baby boomers are the ones dividing up the house and its contents today. The divorce rate for people over age 50 has surged by 50 percent in the past 20 years. Today, one in four of all American divorces involves people over 50.

But here's an interesting twist: By 2009, the divorce rate in the rest of the population began to decline, possibly because people began to marry later and the older couples with young kids were splitting the responsibility for raising the family more evenly, leading to more satisfaction with marriage and the likelihood of stability. Another reason might be the struggling economy and the steep cost of splitting up. Today, about 40 percent of first marriages end in divorce.[9]

The myriad problems faced by 20-somethings during their chaotic search for love and great sex don't end in the 20s—or even with marriage and kids. The perceptions of love and sex formed from what we learned at home and in our teens and 20s leave an indelible mark on us. When teens or 20-somethings have indiscriminate sex with multiple partners, what do they learn about intimacy, love, friendship, and connection? In my opinion, they learn that people are interchangeable and, too often, disposable. I'm all for freedom of choice and having a good time while young and carefree, but I see my patients risking sexually transmitted diseases and disruptive emotional interactions that erode their self-esteem and negatively affect their lives overall. The fact is, every action has consequences regardless what people think when they are 20.

It is very important to remember that at that point in life, sexuality is still hormonally driven. Until the physiological mandate to reproduce is heeded, hormones drive desire, sexual attraction, and lust.

HORMONES: THE INTIMACY CONNECTION

Hormones rule pretty much all actions by 20-something-year-old men and women. The leading driver for sexual activity at this stage remains the pleasure of sex and the biological desire to procreate (primarily for women, not so much for men). Humans need to reproduce in order to keep the species going, and the urge to do so is hardwired into our bodies and minds. Reproduction is in our DNA and the pheromones we disperse into the air around us. No matter the place, time, person, or location, babies must be born. To fulfill this need, we must both have sex *and* attempt to form stable relationships to successfully care for our offspring. The issue for modern women and men is that in order to form a family, you need more than sex, you need a partnership. In general, toward the end of their third decade, both genders start to move away from the notion of sex for sex's sake (even if the move is driven primarily by women).

Unlike other mammals that meet once in order to procreate, and then go about their separate lives, we humans are wired to build our nests and raise our children in the protective crucible of the family or extended family unit. The desire to create a family may appear in women earlier than in men, but by the last few years of the 20s and into the early to mid-30s, it becomes the driving force for most people regardless of gender, cultural background, or social status. While the biological clock is the motivator for women, there is a moment in time when men also start to realize, perhaps subconsciously at times, that they are ready to start their own families. Throughout history, many of our most treasured cultural rituals have been built around these basic desires. While hormones as part of normal human physiology fuel our sexual urges, we also feel an increased need to bond with another person, the father or mother of our children. This bond is also hormonally driven. **Oxytocin** is the hormone of connectivity, and it is released in both women and men when they have an orgasm, when they say they love each other, and especially when a baby is born, firming the bond between mother and child.

Adding to the hormonal pressures are new cultural ones. A lot has changed since the crazy teen years. Twenty-somethings rack up life experience very quickly, modeling themselves after important people in their lives, whether family, friends, or the celebrities they idolize. And whatever these role models do, their followers will do as well.

This is where the question of real *intimacy* returns. Most women are clear that they don't want the father of their babies to be a fly-by-night Lothario, or a man who won't pull his weight in the couple's emotional, financial, and family life. They want someone who will be a shoulder to lean on, a trusted friend and companion to turn to during the rough times—something more than a red-hot lover. If at this point a man or woman learns to separate sex from intimacy, love from lust, he or she can move up to the next level of connection and understanding in human relationships. But because so many 20-somethings still haven't experienced or come to understand what real intimacy means, they keep circling back to the thing they do know—connecting through sex. How do you separate lust from love; heated desire from a meaningful, loving union? For many young people, this is a difficult and often-impassable crossroad. If they continue to equate sex with intimacy, they may spend their entire lives chasing that early sexual high that always fades after the first few months or years when real relationships start to form and must take root or just fail.

Sadly, our media-saturated culture only thwarts our ability to make this crucial leap. We're constantly inundated with tabloid tales of beautiful movie stars who fall in love with their costars on the sets of their romantic dramas and then marry six months later in elaborate fairy-tale weddings. The stars leave behind spouses and children with impunity and without guilt or repercussions. As the blush of passion and romance fades, the couple is left with the same real-life issues they had with previous partners. Meanwhile, publicists help miserable (and mostly unfaithful) celebrity couples maintain the facade of the perfect, loving family and eternally sexually charged relationship. The media shows us the sizzle, but it never offers a glimpse of the steak. That's because there isn't any! The result that I see in my practice is countless starry-eyed women in their 20s, hoping against hope that one late-night hookup will somehow lead them to a happy ending: marriage, children, and a lifetime of loving intimacy. Somehow, that usually happens onscreen more than in real life.

THE EXCEPTION TO THE RULE

While most 20-something relationships are driven by sexual attraction, there are exceptions. Some of those exceptions shed light on sexual problems that affect even young women in their prime.

"My family is very old-fashioned and religious," raven-haired Naomi told me. "A matchmaker introduced my parents, and though their relationship seems horribly boring to me, they say their marriage works. They wanted me to find a husband through a matchmaker as well, and after a series of disastrous dates on my own, I said I'd give it a try. I was matched with the nephew of a man my father works with. We met with both families present, and we were both embarrassed and totally uncomfortable, but over time, we did get to know and learned to like each other. We married three years ago, and last year we had a baby girl. My family is pushing us to have more children, which is expected in our culture. I am so grateful to be married to a good man and to be a new mother, but I don't feel any sexual desire for my husband. What is wrong with me?"

Most likely nothing.

While this may be one of the downsides of arranged marriages, it is a very common complaint in most marriages with the passing of time. Many patients who come from cultures with traditional roles for women and even those from modern backgrounds find themselves torn because the husband is a good provider and often a caring friend and partner, yet no longer (or never was) sexually appealing to them. As time goes by I see more women in these situations, who tell me they never have an orgasm. Too many women still accept that when it comes to enjoying sex, how they feel just doesn't matter that much. But as they watch TV and engage in social media, their world begins to expand and they realize they are missing out on a physiologic right. They are missing out on sexually satisfying lives. While they realize they should be enjoying sex and orgasms, being participants rather than passive observers in the sexual act, they don't know how to get that from their marriages. It's a sociological issue often hard to address and even more difficult to solve.

With the evolution and integration of the various ethnic groups into our melting-pot modern American culture, many marriage issues have become ever more complicated as people from different backgrounds couple up. As each member of the couple brings his or her own cultural biases to the marriage, it becomes imperative to realize it takes a lot of serious and never-ending work to make any marriage work.

While sociological and cultural factors affect relationships and sexuality profoundly during the 20s and 30s, hormone levels remain high and in good balance to help us maintain a strong sexual drive, leading us to reproduce, to fulfill the mission of our existence. Still, there are changes that do occur at every age. In women, before periods, estrogen and progesterone levels drop if the woman doesn't get pregnant, causing bloating and changes in our general mood and sex drive. The female sex drive is the highest around the time of ovulation and right before the period starts. Wanting to have sex before ovulation is physiology at work. Premenstrual syndrome is a mixture of physical symptoms manifesting the drop in hormones that occurs right before a woman gets her period. If PMS is more than a nuisance—if it changes a woman's personality, makes her irritable, and leads to out-of-control food cravings, serious weight gain from water retention, and sleep disturbances—it usually means the hormone balance is not pitch-perfect, but this can easily be helped with additional natural progesterone. I have been successfully treating thousands of women for decades with progesterone before their periods and eliminating PMS.

But it isn't just hormones. Every person is different. As we'll see throughout this book, there are couples in their 70s enjoying great sex, miserable couples in their 30s who haven't had sex in months or even years, and happy couples and singles who don't care about sex at all. Sexuality is very personal, and the key to figuring it out is learning to be honest with yourself. But in general, if an emotionally mature and physically healthy 20-year-old woman has little or no sex drive, something is going on. It could be emotional—as in the case of Naomi and her utilitarian marriage—it could be an issue of low self-esteem, or it could be environmental or due to sleep deprivation, lack of exercise, poor diet, medications like antidepressants and birth control pills, and many other variables contributing to the situation. Nothing should be ignored when trying to get to the root of the problem, and it is very rare that one issue alone causes the problem.

DECREASE IN LIBIDO DURING THE 20S

POSSIBLE CAUSES	POSSIBLE SOLUTIONS
Repressed or overly sexualized upbringing	Seek psychological evaluation and support.
Birth control pills, NuvaRing	Discontinue the pill or take out NuvaRing.
Other medications (antidepressants, blood pressure or ADHD medication, sleeping pills, anti-inflammatories, antibiotics, etc.)	Re-evaluate the need for and use of the medications. Discontinue as soon as possible.

Poor Diet	Eliminate sugar substitutes and fried and processed foods. Reduce alcohol, soda, processed sugar, and caffeine consumption. Eat regular meals made with healthy natural and organic foods.
Lack of sleep	Make sleep a priority with seven to eight hours a night. Make up for lost sleep on weekends.
Stressors from work and personal life	Therapy, coaching, meditation, and regular exercise. Learn to prioritize addressing stressors. Change job if it's destructive to well-being.
Hormone imbalance	Evaluate thyroid, adrenal, estrogen, progesterone, and testosterone balance and treat as needed with bioidentical/natural hormone support.

Depression	Seek talk therapy and increase awareness and self-understanding. (Avoid antidepressant medications in general and specifically those that lower sex drive and change your personality.)
Unsatisfying or abusive relationship	Identify and eliminate abusive relationships from your life. Use coaching and therapy to focus on helping create satisfying and positive relationships. Focus on honesty and building self-confidence. Leave if things don't improve. Never accept abuse or compromise yourself. *Be kind to yourself.*

THE BIRTH CONTROL EFFECT

Birth control pills have been around since the 1930s. Originally developed by a number of scientists, including Carl Djerassi, they were used to sterilize women in Nazi concentration camps during World War II before Margaret Sanger started pioneering its use in the US in the 1950s. Few people know that, including most doctors. By the 1960s, the women's liberation movement turned the pill into a symbol of sexual freedom, equality, and liberation for women. The idea was that if women didn't have to worry about getting pregnant, they could enjoy sex for pleasure the same way men always had.[10]

But there's more to that story.

As we touched upon in the previous chapter, birth control pills are synthetic hormone-like substances that suppress a woman's entire hormone production system, from the pituitary gland (the master gland) in the brain to the thyroid, adrenals, and ovaries. Birth control pills prevent women from having a normal menstrual cycle in which they ovulate and produce estrogen and progesterone—they eliminate the normal female hormone balance. A blood test of hormone levels in a woman on birth control pills will reveal either inappropriately low estrogen and progesterone levels, or even none at all. This means *a woman on birth control pills is operating with the same hormone levels as a woman in menopause.*

As a direct effect of birth control pills, women stop ovulating. That is the mechanism by which birth control pills prevent women from getting pregnant. That's what they are designed to do. Rarely do we hear someone talk about this downside, the fact that the pill doesn't affect just our reproductive organs. It alters the function of every organ in a woman's body while she is on the pill—and after she stops using it.

The body undergoes immediate changes once the pill is started. The many side effects of the pill include mood changes, brain fog, breast enlargement, weight gain, acne, headaches, and loss of sex drive. Over the years, clinicians and researchers have reported and documented many long-term problems that occur from the continuous use of the pill over long periods of time. Since every woman is different, reactions and side effects vary from person to person. Some women can be on the pill for 20 years without noticing anything is wrong. Others, however, suffer with immediate problems like headaches, mood swings, and loss of libido and subsequently develop a higher risk of infertility, blood clots, and certain cancers. All of these side effects make the pill far more dangerous than advertised. Today, gynecologists hand out birth control pills like candy the moment a girl goes into puberty. And as we discussed in Chapter 3, the pill doesn't prevent STDs, which is another highly dangerous aspect and the FDA hasn't approved the pill to regulate periods.

In her book *Sweetening the Pill*, author Holly Grigg-Spall does a great job of describing in detail the truth about the pill and the politics behind its omnipresence in women's lives. She extensively and thoroughly researched the data and has brought to light many of the hidden facts and secret dangers of this female-*un*friendly method of pregnancy prevention.

When a healthy young woman comes to me complaining of little or no sex drive, I do a complete hormone blood panel, then spend as much time as needed to figure out what her family health history contributes and what her diet, sleep, exercise, medication, and supplement programs are, while always paying attention to the details of the stressors and pressures in her life. I find that I spend a lot of time taking women off the pill, NuvaRing, and antidepressants, all of which are common culprits in a young woman's loss of libido, along with many other issues like chronic fatigue, fibromyalgia, depression, anxiety, just to name a few.[11] "The Use of Oral Contraception: A Review of Measurement Approaches." Journal of Women's Health reported troubling findings.[12] The study examined the sexual side effects of birth control pills and other hormonal methods of contraception. Women on birth control methods reported feeling less sexy than women who used a nonhormonal birth control method (intrauterine device, fertility awareness methods, rhythm method, diaphragm, and so forth). The same women also reported fewer orgasms and increased difficulty becoming aroused. Less frequent sex was an obvious side effect. Sadly and oddly, the media often does not cover any of this information even though it is found in the conventional medical literature.

A very popular yet highly dangerous birth control device is the third-generation birth control device known as NuvaRing. This is a ring containing a synthetic progestin called drospirenone, which causes high levels of a hormone-like substance to be released suddenly into the bloodstream, leading to significant increases in the risk of potentially lethal blood clots. A story by Marie Brenner in the January 2014 edition of *Vanity Fair*[13] tells the horrific story of two women in their 20s who used the device and died as a result of blood clots in the lungs. One of the young women, 24-year-old Erica Langhart, died on Thanksgiving Day 2011. Less than a month after her death, a congressional hearing on the safety of third-generation birth control pills and devices, including NuvaRing, kept these dangerous contraception methods on the market despite proven dangers and the deaths they cause. The congressional hearing panel was made up primarily of industry members, and a letter by David Kessler, MD, the former surgeon general, was not accepted as evidence. The letter contained very important information on the dangers of these drugs.

As of this writing, there has been no change in the situation. Special interest groups rule the marketing and information that both women and their physicians are exposed to, and the truth is deeply hidden. As a result, it is practically impossible for young women today to become truly empowered and make safe decisions. The parents of Erica Langhart and many other caring and highly educated people have committed to opening the door on the hidden truth about birth control pills while fighting an uphill battle against the special interest groups that serve to endanger and increase the risks women face every day in this area of their lives. There are safer methods of contraception, like nonhormonal IUDs, FAMs, and certainly condoms, which do not put young women's lives in danger, yet they are less likely to gain more acceptance and use in the present climate. Physician education is lacking, and women don't have the information they need to protect themselves.

SEXUALITY AND YOUR PERSONAL TRUTH

As I mentioned at the beginning of the book, after many years of listening to people and figuring out how to better help my patients accomplish their goals in health, sex, and life, I came to define "personal truth" as an individual's honest way of perceiving and relating to her or his world. When we're young, personal truth emerges from a combination of what we are taught and see at home as well as from friends, formal and informal education, authority figures, and media exposure. Those influences continue to affect us throughout our entire lives. The more sexuality plays a part in our lives from childhood on, the more our perception and interpretation of sex affect our overall behavior. As we move from our 20s into our 30s, our hormonal makeup starts to shift. A solid foundation and a strong sense of who we are become even more crucial as we navigate the choppy waters of sex, marriage, family, commitment, intimacy, and what we would like to believe will be everlasting love and a solid and satisfying family life.

CHAPTER 5

THE COMMITTED
RELATIONSHIP

"The success of marriage comes not in finding the 'right'
person, but in the ability of both partners to adjust to the
real person they inevitably realize they married."
—John Fischer

You finally found each other. And this time, you're sure it's the
real thing. Both of you are truly convinced you are "soul mates."
You share the same likes, dislikes, and life goals. You're on fire
in bed. You tell each other, "I love you," and you feel it to the
core of your very being. Every cell in your bodies aches to be
with each other. Separating even for the day is painful, and
you cannot wait to be together again. Life is all about sharing
everything with each other. Love motivates every step you take
together and apart. You are a team, partners, committed to one
another and to your relationship. So, as a couple, you naturally
make the big decision to spend the rest of your lives together
and build a family. The summer of your sexual life cycle is at

hand from the hormonal and cultural standpoints, but from the relationship perspective, it's autumn on the horizon.

Without a doubt, you believe—and nothing and no one can convince you otherwise—that the life-defining decision you are making is unquestionably correct and solidly backed by the love and passion you feel for each other. All the experiences you have gained from your life so far—experimenting in various previous relationships and one-night stands, even the puppy love of your teens that once seemed the sum of your entire sexual and emotional life—your whole life history has brought you to this momentous decision. It's certainly been a long and winding road so far. You've survived the turbulent transition from an asexual child to a hormone-driven, sex-crazed teen. You suffered through nearly a decade of aimless yet intense sexuality. Motivated primarily by hormones and societal role models, you ran at the speed of light through sequential and even simultaneous sexual experiences with very little connection to emotional development, intimacy, or love.

But now everything has changed. You're in your late 20s to early 30s, and your hormones are beautifully in sync with what society expects of you. You've met the right partner, and starting a family and reproducing will now become your primary life goal.

THE WEDDING-BELL TRAP

Your entire life focus suddenly shifts from the chase, from your fun and commitment-free life as a single person, to the engagement and wedding preparations. In the eyes of both society and your family and friends, you have successfully graduated to the next phase in life. You can now integrate into the social order as an adult, no longer an uninitiated and reckless teen nor a free and easy 20-something. The outside world approves. You are now entering the world as an adult couple.

Even if you and your partner have lived together for years, the dramatic changes that engagement and marriage bring to a relationship are decisive, and they often significantly change the delicate balance between the two of you. Consider the immediate changes: The two of you must now start making very different decisions than before there was a wedding looming in your future. Are you going to tell your family? Are you preparing for an engagement party or a destination wedding? Who will pay for the festivities? How long of an engagement will you have? What are the religious implications of your union? Who will make it onto your invitation list? How involved will you allow your parents to be in the process? The list of questions goes on forever. And speaking of family, now you've got extended family to worry about. Where will you go for Thanksgiving and Christmas or other holidays? Each one of you will have to find ways to integrate your in-laws into your new life, regardless of how you may feel about them. Come to think of it, how will the two sides of your soon-to-be-blended family get along? No matter how well you got along with each other's families before, new issues, changes in involvement, misunderstandings, and arguments will undoubtedly occur once you transition to being a married couple.

Suddenly, all the very small and very large decisions of your life have to take another person into consideration. From the choice of what to eat for dinner to whom you like to spend time with among your family and friends, to the placement of the sofa in the living room, you now have two tastes and opinions to integrate. Then there are the bigger issues to think about, like finances, where to live, the role of religion in your married life, and of course having children. Today, with 47 percent of women in the labor force, the traditional arrangement of man as bread-winner and woman as homemaker has become a thing of the past.[1] Your respective salaries may very well shift the relationship balance. A recent University of Chicago study strongly suggests that many men still aren't comfortable when their wives make more money than they do. In such couples, both the wife and husband generally reported being less happy about the marriage.[2]

All these factors—and many more—will dramatically affect your relationship. I've seen it again and again: A young couple gets so distracted by the bells and whistles of the wedding that, sometimes without realizing it, they shift focus from the two of them—their intimacy and their sexuality—to the planning and implementation of an enormous time- and emotion-consuming undertaking in which it's no longer about the couple but rather the world around them.

"I'm not, and I never thought of myself as someone who follows the crowd," said Christina, a new bride at 28. "So I was surprised and disappointed in myself when I realized I'd been totally sucked into the media hype and craziness around wed-dings. The bridal magazines, the wedding shows on TV, the internet sites—I was practically addicted to Pinterest—it all contributed to the crazy whirlwind that my fantasy wedding day turned into. The unspoken yet loud and strong message I got was, "If the wedding day is flawless, then the rest of your marriage will take care of itself," and I bought into it—hook, line, and sinker. I was determined to make everything perfect. I felt I was in a reality TV show—I didn't want to turn into a 'bridezilla,' but it definitely seemed as though the wedding became the most important thing in my life, and everything else took a back seat, including my relationship with my fiancé.

"My mom and sister went dress shopping with me, and of course I had to have the one that I needed to lose 10 pounds to fit into. I also went overboard picking the perfect dresses for my bridesmaids. I had to be in charge of everything—the invitations, the engagement party, the shower, the rehearsal dinner, down to the tiniest detail. It seemed that suddenly I could no longer focus on anything else in my life. I couldn't sleep, was totally useless at work, and was stressed to the max after spending far more money than my parents, Dave, and I could afford. I was obsessed with losing weight. I dieted and went to bridal boot camp until I'd dropped 20 pounds—10 more than I needed. I didn't recognize myself, but I had no time to do anything different. I just wanted it all to be perfect. I barely noticed, but with the weight and the stress, down went my sex drive.

"Before the planning started, Dave and I used to have sex three to four times a week and more on weekends. Gradually, our sex life just disappeared. Though the wedding itself turned out to be beautiful and a lot of fun for our family and friends, by the wedding night, sex seemed more of an obligation to me. I even felt obligated to slip into the expensive, sexy nightgown I'd received at my bridal shower, even though I was so exhausted that I fell asleep the moment we hit the bed. I think Dave was a little disappointed, but he was burned out from entertaining all day and night too."

And then, there was the honeymoon.

"Your honeymoon is supposed to be your chance for plain, uninterrupted sex and romance after the long buildup to the wedding. It's supposed to be your magical time together as newlyweds. Dave and I were thrilled to be married and have a full week to enjoy each other alone now that we were actually 'legal' and didn't have to worry about protection. But when your expectations are to have sex to top all the sex you've ever had before the wedding, the entire thing turns into more pressure. We went to Hawaii, which is a honeymooner's paradise, so there were hundreds of other couples at the resort along with us. I started to feel weird. I couldn't help but wonder if some of the others were feeling the same. Every morning we all went to breakfast in our beautiful new bathing suits and cover-ups; we spent the day on the beach and went from meal to meal following the same schedule. It was beautiful in spite of my worries, and the time flew by so fast, I felt it was just a dream. And suddenly the entire thing—the preparations, the wedding, and the honeymoon—was over.

"When we got back home to our everyday lives, reality suddenly hit hard. For me, the adjustment was really tough. It was such a letdown. I loved Dave; our relationship was great—so why did I feel so down? Why wouldn't I? After a year of being a bride-to-be, the center of attention, suddenly I was a regular person again. I wasn't so special anymore. I felt bad for Dave, who was patient and kind and didn't understand what was wrong with me. I changed. I lost interest in him, our relationship, and worst of all, sex was never the same for me. I totally lost the passion and spontaneity. I hate to say it, but it became another one of my jobs, like keeping the apartment clean or picking up the clothes from the cleaners—just another chore. Strangely, I'm not the only one feeling this way. Many of my married girl-friends say the same thing. It may start right after the wedding or it may take a few months or even years, but eventually they all say it loses the excitement. What happened?"

Things are always better when they are spontaneous and not forced upon us by outside influences. That's human nature. Adjusting to married life and maintaining the same degree of passion and sexuality we enjoyed before is a tall order. Many of my patients tell me they don't tell the truth about what happens behind closed doors, because they're ashamed and they think friends and family would be disappointed. After all, so much money and effort were poured into the wedding as the ultimate transition to adulthood that no one wants to admit it's not all "happily ever after." According to *Forbes Magazine*, *Huffington Post*, and other media, the wedding and bridal industry is a 40- to 50-billion dollar business catering to approximately 2.5 million couples a year![3] You can certainly understand why it's in the best interest of the wedding industry to sell the myth of the perfect "event" wedding to as many starry-eyed brides and grooms as possible. I try to remind my patients who are brides-to-be that the wedding day will pass in a flash. The goal is to relax and enjoy every moment, to make great memories that will be there forever but to keep things in perspective and not lose sight of their relationships, and to remember that the goal is to build a strong marriage to last a lifetime. Keep yourself and your fiancé front and center and you will enjoy the wedding planning, the wedding, the honeymoon, and your life together.

I'll give you an interesting example of a couple who toned down their expectations for their wedding—and focused on strengthening their relationship instead.

Pete and Mary, both 25, bright, and attractive, met through friends and took their time getting to know each other. After a year of their spending a lot of time together—mostly on their own, becoming friends, enjoying lots of sex, and building a truly intimate relationship—Pete proposed. Their families were thrilled. The couple came from a small town where everyone knew each other, so the entire community was excited by the prospect of the wedding, the parties, and other festivities. Pete's and Mary's parents, grandparents, and siblings were ready to dig in and get involved in planning the wedding of the year.

But Pete and Mary had their own ideas. Despite pressures from her mother and sisters, who were already discussing the details of Mary's wedding, Mary broke the news that she and Pete wanted a simple ceremony. Instead of focusing on elaborate plans, the couple used the year before the wedding to spend even more time alone. They saw movies after work, took cooking classes, or just hung out together. They joined a gym near their apartment and went three times a week after work together. On weekends, they took mini breaks and used the time to deepen their bond. While they felt bad about disappointing their families, ultimately their wedding celebration was small but beautiful and deeply significant to everyone who attended—and most of all, to Mary and Pete. When their wedding night came, they were closer than ever and sex was more passionate than ever and even more intimate. As a plus, they used the money they'd saved by skipping an expensive wedding to take a two-week cruise in the Caribbean. They spent their honeymoon touring new places, relaxing in the sun, and making plans for their future.

Are Pete and Mary more likely to stay married forever? No one has the answer; only time will tell. In their favor are the facts that they come from similar backgrounds, have similar values and life goals, and spent time getting to know each other long before the wedding. A big party and a beautiful dress were less important to them than a strong bond and building a solid foundation for the children they wanted to bring into this world. Their sex life remained terrific maybe mostly because they loved and knew each other so well. They didn't fall into the wedding-bell trap of putting on a show for the outside world. They didn't forget to take care of the two most important people in the marriage.

And, just like Pete and Mary, there are many couples with great intimacy and successful relationships even though they do fall into the wedding-bell trap. They just regroup and adjust to the new life, and pick up where they left off before the nuptials and refocus on each other.

Nothing is permanent and everything can be improved, changed, and recaptured as long as the two people love each other and are intimate and caring. Putting the relationship ahead of the individual ingredients always works. Life is full of change, and the faster the two adjust to change as a couple, the more likely they are to succeed in creating a solid relationship that lasts.

DECISIONS, DECISIONS AND MORE IMPORTANT DECISIONS

Do you want to have a family, or do children not figure into your life plan? Biologically speaking, this is a decision you have to make pretty early on in a committed relationship. To many women, thinking at 25 about having children—when they're barely out of their parents' homes, college, or grad school—seems premature, but the reality is that women's fertility is at its peak until the mid- to late 30s. Though fertility treatments and in-vitro fertilization (IVF)—a two-billion-dollar-a-year booming industry—make it possible for women to conceive well into their 40s, the price is steep and not everyone can afford it both financially and emotionally. Anyone who has gone through it will tell you that, besides being prohibitively expensive, brutal on the body, depressing to the mind, and stressful to the relationship, IVF puts both partners on a long emotional and physical roller coaster that might not even result in conception even though IVF now boasts a success rate of more than 90 percent.[4] It may be harsh, unfair, and cruel, but it is a *fact*: You and your partner need to be on the same page with regard to having children, and You need to figure out where you stand on this topic sooner rather than later.

My recommendation is to talk about it before you get married.

NOT EVERY PERSON FITS THE MOLD

At the beginning of this book, I stressed that it's our individuality that defines us as people, and in time we figure out who we truly are as sexual beings, even though we live in a society that tries its best to squeeze us all into the same mold regardless of what stage of life we're in. As I spend time listening to patients, I'm often struck by the way young people robotically choose life goals that follow a predetermined path toward marriage and children, often without considering what they personally might need to feel complete and happy. Too many women—and even some men—who don't succeed in finding a mate or don't get married by 30 tell me they are embarrassed, become desperate, and feel like failures. Those who simply don't aspire to marriage and family are viewed by society as pariahs—asexual or unwilling to admit they are gay. All this may sound old-fashioned, but sadly it's true even today. This may be why so many young people let a lukewarm relationship snowball into a wedding, followed too often by an unhappy, emotionally disappointing, and frustrating marriage. They do it because they're afraid to let their families down, they're ashamed and dread being viewed as different by the world around them, and they just don't want to be alone in a society in which each person is expected to be part of a couple. This is a tragedy we must undo in our lifetime.

Having listened to hundreds of patients who've shared with me the consequences of unwise and poorly thought-out choices, I must stress that this is your life and:

No matter how much pressure you might feel from our culture, your family, and your friends, there are no guarantees that following the path of others will make you happy or even guarantee you a fulfilled life. There is no such thing as right or wrong in sexuality, intimate relationships, and personal life choices. To be successful, these things must be personal.

I cannot stress enough that *we are all unique, with unique needs.* As our society evolves, we must become more accepting and less judgmental. It is the kinder, better message that behooves a civilized society to live by.

Jill, a stunning honey blonde actress, was 40 by the time she realized she had been looking for the right guy for far too many years. When she was in her 20s and men flocked to her, she figured she had plenty of time. Opportunities kept presenting themselves and, enhanced by her career status and beauty, Jill never missed the chance to party and have sex with many charming and attractive guys. But she always found flaws in her numerous suitors. No one, it seemed, was good-looking, successful, smart, or rich enough.

Just like many other women in her situation, Jill secretly hoped that every new man she slept with would turn into the prince of her own personal romance novel after a few evenings together. Eventually, she was sure, the plot would play out predictably with his marrying her and sweeping her away on his private jet or yacht. When that didn't happen by her late 20s, she became serially monogamous. Yet all the guys she went out with cheated on her, leaving her doubting her own judgment and unclear about how to choose the right one. Seeking answers, she started therapy and quickly faced her previously hidden emotional issues. Her father had cheated on her mother, and Jill was the one in the family who had found out, when she was barely a teen. She had told her mother, who wouldn't think of leaving her father. Instead, the mother pretended her marriage was the model of the ideal relationship. She taught both her daughter and son that their parents' less-than-honest union was okay and the only way to live life in an acceptable manner.

As the years passed, Jill became desperate to find the right guy. But that isn't how she presented it to the outside world. She vacillated between convincing herself—and anyone who would listen—that she wanted a huge movie career and, conversely, that she just wanted to retire from show business altogether, settle down, and start a family. Since she never honestly owned what she really wanted, she kept attracting, and being attracted to, men who did not commit to her. Her life was a constant roller coaster of drama. By the time Jill realized that her issues with relationships with men weren't going away, her biological clock was seriously ticking away. Panic set in, and her obvious desperation and fear started to make her unappealing to men in general. Eventually, in her mid-40s, Jill did fall in love and settled down with a kind man with children from a previous marriage, while her career fizzled. To this day, she still struggles with regrets about both her career and her unfulfilled desire to have carried her own children.

Although I hear stories like Jill's far too often, women can avoid her predicament when they're comfortable and honest with themselves and are able to put their lives in honest perspective. Everyone can make career and family choices early on and still feel free to change his or her mind as life takes unexpected turns. Having supportive parents who are honest and don't give mixed messages or deceive their kids is important, but as we get older, it is our personal responsibility to figure out what we want out of our lives and careers. We can't blame our parents forever for the mistakes we make in our lives.

In my experience, there are many Jill types on career paths in the corporate fast lanes of big cities. I see too many women in early menopause either realizing it's too late to have children or still trying after as many as 20 IVF courses. They are unhappy, and not only because they didn't have children or aren't married to the perfect guy. Mostly, they are unhappy because they did not make their own decisions earlier in life.

In the early 2000s, I was on a TV show called *Scarborough Country*, hosted by Joe Scarborough. The segment I appeared on addressed the biological time clock, and I was one of two guests. The other guest was a journalist who had written an article on the topic for *The Washington Post*, warning professional women that they were in danger of finding themselves childless if they didn't watch their biological clock. As both a professional woman and mom myself, I wanted to give women hope and empower them. I was afraid the journalist was there to limit women's options.

But as the segment unfolded, I realized the journalist and I were saying the same thing. For women, the biological clock just keeps ticking. Unless they pay attention, too many find themselves at 50 with a highly successful career and no children, or with no career and with children grown and out of the house, and no prospects for work in the field they abandoned decades earlier. How do we help women navigate these muddy and rough waters? Men don't have this problem, which I suspect causes much of the disparity in career decisions and life outcomes for men and women, even in our newly evolved so-called egalitarian society.

WHERE DO YOU FIT IN?

Both women and men in cities are waiting longer before getting married. The average age women and men marry in the United States has risen consistently over the past 50 years. In 1960, the average age for a woman to get married was 20 and for a man was 22. Compare that with the averages today: 27 for women and 29 for men.[5]

For women, it appears that the more money they earn, the longer they wait to marry. The highest-earning women are those over 30 with a college degree who don't seem to jump into getting married. In contrast, education doesn't matter as much for men. Regardless of degree men who marry in their late 20s earn more money than those who marry earlier.

Where earning potential is concerned, women benefit from marrying later, while for men the opposite is true. Doesn't that directly counter the imperative of women's biological clocks?

WHAT'S LOVE GOT TO DO WITH IT?

What does "love" mean?

At different ages, "love" means different things. Mothers and fathers can't take their eyes off their newborn. This is love. Friends show their love for one another through loyalty and support. Most family members, even those who bicker, are there for one another regardless of how they might choose to express it. Teens, lost in a hormonal fog, express their love in a number of ways, including sexualizing it and confusing it with intimacy. Adults form loving bonds that take many different forms and meanings.

And, of course, there's the love we read about in Valentine's Day cards, the romantic definition of "love" that fuels novels, movies, and mostly fantasies. In this version, being in love with another person means that we are so wrapped up in our emotions and desire to spend all our time with the other person that we tune everything and everyone else out. Sexual love is usually associated with passion, the desire for sex, and exclusivity—when men and women decide they no longer will have sex with other people.

When two people get married and profess exclusivity to each other, they usually do so out of love. However, for many 20- to 30-year-olds, love is a complex combination of lust, passion, connection, intimacy, common interests, desire, and exclusivity. The story of "who said 'I love you' first" in young relationships often determines the transition from casual to serious exclusive relationships. Often uttered during or after sex, "I love you" to some means, "I want to be with you sexually, emotionally, possibly leading to a committed relationship." But since the term "love" is so confusing and broad, people don't always know or understand the nuances associated with these three little, life-altering words. Once uttered, these three words immediately alter the perception of the course of the relationship. That is quite powerful!

Yet at the same time, we live in a society in which "I love you" is very casually thrown around. We get off the phone saying, "Love you," to friends or even acquaintances when we really mean, "I like you and wish you a nice day." We say, "I love you," to friends, family, kids, and—undoubtedly with total sincerity—to our pets. So why, then, does saying, "I love you," in a romantic setting have an entirely different meaning than in our daily lives? Why do we expect commitment to an exclusive relationship when "I love you" is said in a sexual relationship?

THE MONOGAMY QUESTION

Are humans meant to be monogamous? How do we know?

Let's take a look at the animal kingdom. Monogamy is rare among mammals. The classic example of monogamy in mammals is the little prairie vole, a rat-like creature that chooses one partner early; bonds, mates, and nests with that partner; raises the young; and stays with that partner for life. The prairie vole is clearly monogamous. One partner for life. Well, that is if the aforementioned activities represent the definition of monogamy. You noticed that I skipped sexuality. That is because prairie voles aren't sexually exclusive. Over the course of their monogamous lives, they have a few discreet sexual trysts to break up the monotony.[6] Yep, the monotony of one sex partner for life. Because, no matter what our culture tells us to believe, things do get monotonous after a while.

Among the most social mammals—from wolves to elephants to dolphins—sexual relationships are complex, often more like the communal arrangements of polygamous cultures. For instance, wolf packs are built around two wolves, the alpha male and female, that sometimes do mate for life but are sexually active with each other only once a year, during breeding season. The other wolves in the pack aren't allowed to mate, but help raise the pups. Outwardly, the male and female wolves appear monogamous, but a closer look reveals the fact that every so often, their relationship becomes an "open marriage"—on some occasions, the female alpha will breed with another male in the group, or the male alpha with another female, perhaps to add to the pack's numbers and, most likely, to diversify their gene pool—and maybe to break up the monotony.[7]

A wolf pack is basically a family unit. Like tribal or traditional cultures, social mammals live in extended families, so they don't need to be monogamous—the whole group, particularly the females, helps with raising the young. Deeply felt group bonds and loyalty in societies like those of whales or dolphins seem to take the place of what we know as "romantic" love. These creatures may be as deeply and emotionally devoted to one another as we are to our mates, but it's more a social than a sexually exclusive devotion.

Monogamy itself seems to have evolved in the later centuries of primate evolution, where it's estimated that 27 percent of species (as opposed to 9 percent of mammals as a whole) practice some sort of "social monogamy."[8] Scientists have been arguing for decades about exactly why and how monogamy came about. Was it because it prevented infanticide by rival male primates, who didn't want to be stuck raising another male's young? Were males simply *forced* into monogamy because females of their species spread out over too wide a geographical area, making it impossible for a horny primate male to juggle multiple girlfriends at once? Overall, everyone agrees that monogamy ended up giving primates—and humans—a real evolutionary advantage.[9] "Pair bonding" in groups where a male protects his offspring long enough for the offspring to make it to adulthood means the survival of the species is far more likely. Since primate infants develop more slowly and need longer-term care, having the male around longer is welcomed.[10] The bonding that takes place during that time appears to be the evolutionary predecessor to married coupling and love.

However, social monogamy in primates doesn't necessarily mean sexual faithfulness. Though both sexes are known to stray, males in particular seem driven to find other opportunities to hook up. Let's take our fellow primate, the gibbon, as an example. Like the prairie voles, male and female gibbons pair up, mate, and nest together monogamously, sometimes for many years at a time. The males always stick around to raise their young—but, once in a while, they'll stray into another female's territory and have sex with her. This may—or may not—result in a "divorce" from the primary partner.[11]

Most anthropologists agree that monogamy, with all its advantages, came at a very late stage in primate evolution and was a later development in human societies as well. That means our biological wiring is likely still more like that of the gibbon—or even of our closest primate relative, the highly promiscuous chimpanzee. This points to the possibility that monogamy is culturally—not biologically—imposed. Even today, more than 60 percent of "traditional" societies allow men to have more than one wife. Monogamy may be an evolutionary advantage, but the latest science and our own experience tell us that, as humans, we're still getting used to the concept.[12]

STAYING FAITHFUL

Clearly, our relatives in the animal kingdom are not promising their mates eternal devotion, and neither were our homo sapiens ancestors. Does that mean we're just brainwashed to believe "happily ever after" exists and monogamy is feasible in a long marriage?

When we are in our 20s and 30s, many of us believe that exclusivity and monogamy are naturally expected, and, should a partner breach them, they are deal breakers. To believe we are loved, to love with abandon, to trust, to passionately idolize our partners—at this point in our lives, this adds up to implied and explicit sexual fidelity. Most American women and men would not agree to commit to another person if, like our primate relatives, they were willing to accept their partners' sexual indiscretions as just a fact of life.

But once commitment and real life set in, the perspective changes. Life is a series of phases, and in each phase, we gain a different perspective and insight into ourselves, our interactions with the outside world, and the significance and importance of our sexuality and its connection to intimacy.

"When Joe and I got married five years ago, I was so happy," Elisabeth, 36, told me. "It all happened very quickly. We met on a plane—as it happened, on the way to the same conference. We found ourselves staying at the same hotel, and we ended up meeting for dinner every night. We flirted a lot from the start, and on the last night of the conference, we ended up in his room having sex and spent the night together. We had the best sex ever. We agreed to keep seeing each other when we got home, and we did. A few months later, Joe asked me to marry him, and I was happy to say yes. My mother told me that getting to know someone takes a lifetime, so I figured that's what we would do. It wasn't as if we were starting from zero. After all, we were in the same line of business, played tennis, enjoyed sport events, and joined a wine club together, not to mention we spent all our free time in bed having amazing sex.

"For the first couple of years, everything was great between us. And then something shifted; it's hard to pinpoint when it happened. Maybe it was the sameness of our everyday lives that wore us down. On weekdays, waking up at the same time every day and going to work, coming home late and making dinner, cleaning up afterwards, checking emails, working out, and so forth. By the time all the chores were done, it was time to go to sleep. We stopped having sex in the morning, and over time we stopped having sex in the evening too. On weekends, we would see friends or family, get the laundry done, clean the house, go grocery shopping, run errands, and work out. It wasn't as if we fought; we didn't. On the other hand, we didn't talk a lot either. When we went on vacation, we planned a lot of sightseeing. We did have more sex then, but it seemed weird. There wasn't a lot of "us alone" sex time anymore. Over the course of a couple of years, we stopped having sex altogether. When I asked him why, he would shrug his shoulders and say he was tired, or "not feeling up to it." There were all kinds of lame excuses. I should have realized something was off, but I really didn't feel that interested anymore either, and so I just ignored it. I thought it was just normal as our marriage settled in that sex was no longer going to be that important to either one of us.

"Then one day, out of curiosity, I looked at Joe's emails and that's when everything changed. There were porn sites and messages back and forth between him and other women. They were all about sex; some totally explicit, while others heavy teases full of sex talk. When I confronted him, he said that he needed some excitement in his life and saw no harm in what he called "light" porn. It wasn't as if he was actually sleeping with these women, he said, as if that were acceptable. I was so angry and hurt, I stormed out of the house and walked around our neighborhood for a while. I didn't want to call my mom or friends, because I was afraid they would confuse me even more. As I kept walking, I started to admit to myself that I was bored too. But I wasn't interested in porn sites and messages from strangers. I honestly am not sure what I want. Maybe the truth is, I want romance forever even though it's difficult to sustain when you are married for a long time and sex with the same person totally loses its excitement. But then what do I do? My husband chose porn sites, and I chose to ignore the obvious fact that we no longer even tried to have sex. Neither solution seems to help keep our relationship exciting or just simply together. Is there even a possibility of keeping the fires burning in a long-term relationship?"

How unusual is this story? Sadly, it's a common one my patients tell me. I hear variations of it very often. Sex and romance go stale even in solid marriages. Then, either one or both partners might seek sexual excitement in ways that veer off the conventionally acceptable path. Internet pornography and fantasy chatrooms are available at the touch of a keypad. Women and men advertise on Craigslist looking for threesomes, wife swaps, or other outside-the-box sexual encounters. Nobody wants to talk about how many "average" couples participate—and there aren't many studies on how happy those people feel about what they're doing either. When sex goes stale, does going outside the marriage for sex help or hurt? Whether it's a fantasy relationship in cyberspace, an afternoon tryst with a next-door neighbor, wife swapping, threesomes, or business escapades where "what happens in Vegas, stays in Vegas," can turning to alternative methods of sexual satisfaction help revive a dead marriage? Or does infidelity of any kind automatically destroy the already delicate fabric of this tenuous institution?

> ## MARRIAGE SEX STATISTICS[13]
>
> - 44 percent of married couples say they are "fully satisfied" with their sex lives.
> - More than 50 percent of married people older than 65 have sex more than once a week.
> - 39 percent of married people are looking for more love and romance in their marriage.
> - 36 percent of married people would like more quality time with their partner.

IDENTIFYING AND COMMUNICATING YOUR NEEDS

Unless you truly know yourself and spend time developing honest insights into your own needs, you can't communicate those needs to your partner. And unless you are willing to sit down with your partner and face the facts with honesty and deal with a lot of things that are hard to talk about, you cannot improve a relationship or develop true intimacy.

People stray for many reasons, but foremost among them are lack of communication and unreasonable expectations of what marriage should be. In our modern world, most people who get married start out with sexual attraction and lots of sexual activity. But once the honeymoon is over, as time passes and the sexual spark inevitably diminishes, many couples stay silent about their changing relationships. It's not always just the lack of sex that destroys intimacy—I'd argue it's the inability and unwillingness to *talk* about the lack of sex that does most of the damage! Denial, anger, blame, and silence never bring a couple closer. Instead, both partners move further and further apart without admitting or discussing their needs, further diminishing intimacy and communication—vital elements in keeping a relationship alive.

Remember: Sex is not the *same* as intimacy. Sex can be *one* way to express passion, love, and intimacy, best used when we are young, when our hormones are in balance and our sex organs are in peak operating condition. Otherwise, sex is a combination of the drive to procreate and a basic way to relieve stress, like eating when you are hungry and sleeping when you are tired. In our complicated society, we have artificially inflated sex's importance and connection to intimacy, leading to much confusion and leaving too many people at a loss in their quests for loving relationships.

SOLUTIONS

If sex in your committed relationships becomes a source of confusion rather than a pleasure, address it:

- Become real partners—become friends.
- Don't lie, and don't deny. The truth will always set you free no matter how difficult it is to tell.

- Don't give up on the marriage, and don't give up on your ability to make it work. Look at your own actions first.
- Become truly intimate by sharing feelings honestly. Care about your partner's stories.
- Don't look outside the marriage for solutions until you've exhausted all options within the marriage. Let me repeat that: Don't look outside the marriage. Once you break it, it's likely to be permanently damaged.
- Don't be afraid of hurting your partner's feelings by telling the truth. Without the truth, the marriage is doomed anyway. You owe it to yourselves to see if you can work things out.
- Go to marriage counseling if you can't just sit down and talk to each other honestly and kindly.
- Spend time learning to accept each other for who you are today, not the fantasy you have about how you were when you first got together.
- Marriage is constant work. If you don't work on it, it doesn't work. You both will change in time, and unless you change together, you change apart.

CHAPTER 6

YOUNG AND SUDDENLY SINGLE AGAIN

"A season of loneliness and isolation is when the caterpillar gets its wings. Remember that next time you feel alone."

—Mandy Hale

Rebecca realized she'd made a terrible mistake about three years into her marriage to Derek.

"I was only 24, right out of grad school and in my first job at a brokerage firm, when my mother suddenly died. Her death demolished me and my world. When I was grieving her, I felt so alone—my friends in my age group couldn't even imagine losing a parent so young, except for Derek, who was actually my first boss. He was 35, made great money, and it seemed like he had it all together. His father had died a year before my mom did, and he really empathized with me, and our shared grief brought us close together. He was my support through those horrific months right after my mother's passing, and we became more than just friends very quickly. The truth is, our sex life was never the greatest—he didn't like foreplay or even kissing me—but because I was so depressed for two years after I lost my mom, I didn't have much sex drive to begin with. I was just so grateful for his solid and caring shoulder to cry on, I had sex with him whenever he wanted, and I did feel better once in a while when I had an orgasm. I moved in with him within six months, and a year later, we were married. We had a fancy, expensive wedding, and Derek bought us a big house in the suburbs.

"What I didn't realize through the fog of my grief was that subconsciously, I must have been looking for a parent, not a partner…and that's what I ended up with: the parent from hell. The moment we moved to the suburbs, Derek got very controlling. He didn't want me spending time with my friends from school or even having lunch with the other junior brokers at work. He started to get jealous of any guy I spoke to, from the guy at the next trading desk to my dentist. He actively did things to isolate me and kept a tight watch on where I went and every penny I spent. As I finally came out of mourning, my sex drive returned, but oddly, now Derek didn't seem that interested in me. All he would do was criticize everything I did and constantly put me down. I wanted to feel young and have fun again, but all he seemed to care about was work, making money, and keeping me under his thumb. Most nights he would work late and then just go to sleep without even talking to me.

"When I turned 29, I started to think about having kids. But the idea of bringing them into this world with a controlling workaholic for a father was something I couldn't get my head around. I could barely take his negativity and criticisms of me, so how could I consciously bring an innocent child into the home environment I lived in? I knew I couldn't stay with him and the only option was to get out while I was still young and could start over. It wasn't that easy, though. It took two years for me to get the courage to move out, then two more years for the divorce to go through—Derek did his best to drag it out, working hard to make me go broke in the process. Now I'm 34, and though I still dream of a family, I'm burned out, really exhausted, and scared. I don't trust my judgment in men, and I'm terrified I'll be put in a cage again if I allow a guy too close, so I work really long hours and go home alone at night. All I wanted was someone to love me and see me through the hardest time of my life. But now I totally understand, I never should have made the decision to marry at such a vulnerable time."

Hindsight is 20/20.

When young people couple up and stop hooking up just for fun, a shift in their perception and expectations of life occurs. Getting engaged and married is their transition into adulthood. It's not just something that society expects and encourages biologically; it's also the drive to perpetuate the species and to leave something of ourselves behind for the next generation. When we look at our children, we see pieces of ourselves. We see our immortality in their eyes, their hands, their gestures…infinite details. They are an opportunity for a do-over, trying to be the people we hoped to become had our lives turned out differently.

When we become part of a couple in the summer of our sexual lives, most of us don't think about deep and far-reaching consequences. Most of us don't plan on becoming single ever again. We go through the process of dating, getting engaged and married, making a home, making friends, and becoming part of a community of people of similar ages and with similar interests and goals. We take it for granted that this will be forever. Most people don't get married—or fall in love—with the idea that those feelings and decisions are a temporary phase in their lives. And society helps us perpetuate the idea of permanence by reinforcing again and again that creating a unit as a couple—and then as a family—is the only way to go through life the right way. Unfortunately, we have no control over what happens in our lives beyond how we react and how we behave ourselves. It takes many years and making lots of mistakes to get that lesson.

Watching and listening to my patients for decades, I have heard story after story about young people who get into relationships thinking they've got it all figured out, then finding themselves suddenly alone as a result of divorces, tragedies, or other twists of fate that no one could have expected. It would be nice if we all were told the truth. Life is stranger and less predictable than any book, TV show, or movie. Life has no script for us to follow.

WHEN THE UNEXPECTED HAPPENS

Cindy's heart-wrenching story about her brief marriage to Ian, while thankfully unusual, is so terrifying and sad it puts the unpredictability of life into perspective. It also may help us adjust our expectations and become kinder and gentler to each other in general.

"Ian and I went to high school together and fell madly in love the second we met. We grew up living on the same street and our siblings were friends, yet it took us until junior year in high school to notice each other. Once our romance started, we quickly became inseparable. We were both virgins and 16. We learned about sex from videos, talking to friends, the internet and, of course, just trying it out. We went to school together and then home to wherever we could find a private space, and just made out and made love for as long as we could get away with it. It's a miracle I didn't get pregnant.

"In time, with our parents' blessing, we planned our wedding after we both finished high school. Ian planned to go to trade school, and I was going to get a job in an office and, hopefully, quickly become a young mother. Our wedding was beautiful, and our families paid for us to go on a romantic honeymoon to Florida. We never left the bedroom the entire week. All we wanted to do was make love and enjoy each other.

"About six months after we got married, Ian woke up in the middle of the night with a terrible headache. It was so bad we had to go to the hospital. At first, the doctors couldn't figure out what was wrong, and they just gave him painkillers and sent him home. But the headache never went away; it got worse and we went back to the hospital, where he was admitted and had lots of tests. Ian was diagnosed with a blood vessel problem, something like a bubble that burst—bleeding inside his brain. Not long after that, he went into a coma. It all happened so fast. I spent the entire time sitting by his bedside, hoping and praying he would come back to me. He didn't. He died three weeks later. I was a widow at 19.

"It took months for me to even believe he was gone. I was lost—couldn't work, couldn't sleep or eat, just waded through life like through cement. I went into therapy, grief counseling, group therapy, and still I spent every night crying myself to sleep. My therapist wanted to send me to a psychiatrist to take antidepressants, but I didn't want to go that route. *What's the use? I'm not sick. I am mourning, and I am depressed for good reason,* [I thought]. I lost my appetite and 20 pounds within a month of Ian's passing. I went back to work after six weeks and moved back in with my parents.

"It's now been five years since Ian passed. Life is getting better. I'm back in my own apartment; I go out with my girl-friends sometimes. I work full-time. Everyone around me is married and having kids, and some are complaining about their marriages and even getting divorced already. I get so angry with them, because I wish I had the chance to get to hate Ian. It would have been so much easier. People don't realize how losing your husband like that makes him look like he was perfect forever. I haven't had sex since he died, and I doubt I will ever meet another man to take his place. I know he can't be replaced, and I see myself alone for the rest of my life."

Cindy's story is heartbreaking, and there is no way to ratio-nalize what happened to her. She has no other healthy option but to go through the process of mourning, which may take many years before she feels strong enough to open her heart again to meeting the right guy. Knowing what a lovely person she is, I don't believe she will be alone forever, but the solution isn't to push her into a relationship before she is ready for it or give her antidepressants to dull her feelings. As long as she is functional and goes to work and stays connected to her family and friends, it is better for her to feel her profound sadness and pain and let time heal the wound, rather than numbing herself with meds or jumping into bed with other men. The side effects and risks of those options are far more dangerous than her mourning her enormous loss.

DIVORCE HAPPENS TOO

While the divorce rate is dropping for those in first marriages, a large number of young marriages still do end. Divorce is the leading cause of becoming single again during the 20s and 30s, ahead of the death of a partner.[1] Monica and Max are reminders that marrying the wrong person throws a person's life into chaos and confusion.

Monica and Max were both 20 when they met in college, at a football party. They were immediately attracted physically and had sex the first night they met. At breakfast the next morning, they started to talk and learn a bit about each other. It turned out that Max and Monica came from different states and very different family backgrounds. Monica came from New England, and her parents were teachers who believed in the value of education and discipline. She had grown up in a household that was very regimented, strict, and rigid, lacking in emotional warmth and communication. Max, on the other hand, came from California. His parents were hippies, he proudly told Monica, and he was raised in an open atmosphere where no topic was off-limits and his parents talked about their sex life openly. They even allowed him to smoke marijuana at 12, and they never closed their bedroom door when he was growing up. The only rules in his household were to follow your heart, try to save the world, and do whatever you wanted—as long as it didn't hurt others. Max was raised to feel free, while Monica was raised to follow rules.

Despite their differences—or maybe because of them—the chemistry between Monica and Max grew more electric as they learned more about each other. It was a case of opposites attracting—a phenomenon we all live with that often shapes our romantic choices when we are young. From the very start, the two spent every moment together. They studied and ate together, and within a week of meeting, they moved into Max's dorm room. They were passionate and ecstatic about their love affair. Monica laughed as she remembered how Max would ask her to lie on the bed naked, claiming it "helped him study better." Of course, it was more likely to lead to sex than studying. In fact, Monica admitted years later, everything they did in those days led to sex. Since sex was what they lived and breathed during those early passionate years, she was surprised they even graduated.

After college, Max and Monica got engaged and then married, and moved to New England to be near her parents, who were older and needed help.

When Monica came to see me as a patient for the first time, she told me the reason she married Max was that, "he was so sexy, and he came from a carefree background so different from mine, I felt he was my missing piece, the balance to my upbringing and to me as a person." Monica and Max had two children within five years after they got married. They both found good jobs and were able to buy a nice home close to her parents, who, because of their remote, unemotional behavior, never really influenced or interfered with the dynamic of their relationship.

In time, the very differences that brought the couple together caused them to fall apart. Raising children plus shopping and cooking and cleaning for her aging parents, as well as working full-time, were hard on Monica. She was always tired, and over time she grew short-tempered. Max felt resentful because Monica's focus was always on the kids and her parents. And no matter how much time and effort Max put into helping with the kids, the house, and the chores, it was never enough for Monica, who only created more rules and put more demands on him.

The first thing to go from the relationship was the sex. Monica's exhaustion depleted her emotionally, and that was reflected in her flagging sex drive. By the time their second child was born, the couple's sex life had become a fading memory. Getting into bed at night, Max would lament, "was like lying down next to an iceberg, and it had nothing to do with the room temperature." Max could not believe the woman of his dreams, the highly sexed girl Monica had been when they first met, had turned so cold.

To their credit, Max and Monica decided they needed couples therapy and went to get help. There, they were told their predicament was not unusual. Most married couples go through a rough patch in the middle of the marriage, during the time their kids are young, the parents are aging, and their priorities dramatically change from being focused on each other to being focused on everyone and everything else.

That explanation did not help Max. He wanted his fun, sexy wife back, and according to him, she was becoming more rigid—and frigid—with every passing day. Max saw no upside to the relationship for him, and he started staying away from home whenever possible to avoid Monica's constant haranguing and criticism, hanging out late after work at the local bar with his buddies or just finding excuses to not face his wife. Monica took this as proof that Max didn't care and had given up on the marriage. Regardless of what the therapist gave them to do as homework, Monica and Max were unable to implement it as the marriage kept crumbling. They could not break the blame cycle and were barely communicating. Monica felt she had too much responsibility, and Max felt he wasn't loved and appreciated in his own home. Both felt alone, and neither could conjure up the memories of the past to help them talk and bring them back together.

After a few years of trying to make it work unsuccessfully, Max, a hot-blooded sexual man, started to see other women. He later said he was seeking someone—anyone—who would smile and laugh and find him sexy again. He said the lack of sex in the marriage made him crazy, and he became obsessed with figuring out how to get sex. He wanted to be noticed, and Monica had long banished him from her visual field. Eventually, he stopped hiding his affairs from Monica, who threw him out of the house. Both were relieved instead of devastated. The children fared better without the cold war in their home. Once Max was out, Monica's parents moved in with them. Divorce quickly followed.

Monica met a man at work with three kids from his first marriage, and within six months of the divorce from Max, she remarried. Max remarried as well, but only after five more years of playing the field and having sex with, he boasted, "literally a hundred different women." He took his time because, he said, he wanted to make up for the years of being "in jail," which is how he described his marriage to Monica.

Sadly, neither could recall how they felt when it all started, or why their once passionate love affair turned to mutual blame and contempt bankrupting the marriage.

I hear variations on Monica and Max's story a lot. People fall in lust but never really connect sex with true intimacy or develop a really committed relationship. If they can move beyond the sexual fantasy of the early phases of the relationship and grow up into mutually respectful adults able to accept each other, notice each other, and work out compromises, things may work out. If not, the system breaks down and the outcome is a broken marriage whether they stay together for the sake of the kids or just split up.

WHY DO MARRIAGES END? [2]

In 1992, Washington University psychologist John Gottman, PhD, and colleagues set out to discover if they could identify and predict the most common factors that made a couple likely to divorce. Many years and several studies later, Gottman and his psychotherapist wife founded the Gottman Institute, a not-for-profit organization dedicated to couples therapy based on his published findings.[3]

Gottman identified what he calls "The Four Horsemen"—the likeliest communication styles between couples that tend to doom a marriage. They are:

- Criticism
- Defensiveness
- Stonewalling
- Contempt

Gottman and his colleagues also identified the most likely reasons for divorce and the number of years into a marriage divorces were most likely to occur for those reasons:

- Five to seven years, due to high conflict
- Ten to twelve years, due to loss of intimacy and connection

Keep in mind that, even with love and communication at the core of a relationship, the high-energy sparks of sex will fade or at least change in time. That is not necessarily what dooms the marriage. When there is no intimacy—no connection, love, and communication—is when the partners are left alone inside an institution that may have been reduced to a label. Unless they've been preparing together and working through the different phases and stages of marriage, too many couples stay together just because they see no other options.

Linda was 22 when she met Brian, also 22, on a blind date. They liked each other from the first words uttered, and they each felt they had found the right one immediately. The connection was passionate, and they moved in together within a few months. As a couple, they shared an active sex life but no real life goals. They were both busy graduate students with no desire to get married while still in school. After they got their advanced degrees, they both found good jobs. They lived together for eight years until family pressures got to be too much for them. Both Linda's and Brian's parents disapproved of their living arrangement's dragging on so long without a ring. Ultimately, they gave in and decided to get married. Years later, Linda talked about the moment she knew she had made a mistake.

"I knew things had changed and we were suddenly moving in the wrong direction. The evening we were married, we walked into the honeymoon suite and I saw the bed covered with rose petals. It was such a beautiful and romantic sight. But something felt strange to me. Instead of being thrilled, I felt overwhelmed and trapped. Everything flowed naturally before the wedding;

Brian and I had been a team for almost a decade, and no one had to tell us to stay together. We were fine with our life the way it had been. For the first time ever, I asked myself, "Is this the guy I really want to grow old with?" Suddenly the answer was, "I'm not sure." I tried to tell Brian how I felt. He was drunk and happy and oblivious to my panic, wanting to just get into bed and have sex. I felt paralyzed; for the first time in our relationship I didn't want sex—I wanted to run away. Instead, I got into bed and…I faked it. On the honeymoon we had sex every day, though I no longer enjoyed or looked forward to having it the way I used to. I noticed that faking orgasms did not make any impact on Brian. He seemed oblivious to the change in me. I used to think he got me, he totally knew me so well, and here I was faking it and he had no idea. I knew then I didn't love him anymore.

"We stayed married for three years, but things went from bad to worse. It got so [bad] that I couldn't stand the sight of him. Brian either didn't notice—which I can't really believe—or he was in complete denial, which only made things worse. I kept trying to reach out to him, but something held me back. I grew sullen and he didn't seem to notice that either. Now all I did was pick on all the things I thought were wrong with him. Things that didn't matter before—like his being sloppy and my being a neat freak, him leaving the toilet seat up or forgetting to buy the specific brand of paper towels I asked for—all became excuses for never-ending bickering and more dead space between us. I fell out of love with him to the point I even dreaded meeting him for dinner. I knew this was all wrong, but I didn't know how to change it. Or maybe I just didn't want it to change. The thought of sex with him turned me off, and I came up with all kinds of excuses to avoid it: headaches, work, periods, friends in need of help—anything. But I couldn't talk to any of my family or friends, because in front of them we acted like everything was great and I was too embarrassed to tell them otherwise. I hoped that if we put on a good face, our life behind closed doors would somehow catch up. I don't know what I was thinking. It was crazy.

"And Brian? He thought it was just a phase I was going through. I have no idea how he thought things would get better without us ever talking about it or acknowledging there was a problem. Strangely, one day he started talking about starting a family. His parents had been telling him that having children was a sure way to keep our marriage together, and he thought having a child was what I surely wanted. For me that was the straw that broke the camel's back. How could he be so unaware of what was going on between us?

"I asked him to go for marriage counseling with me. Brian refused to go at first, because he said I was the one who thought there was a problem. But my boss, a twice-divorced friend in her 40s who had gone through the same thing in her first marriage, told me she thought counseling might have saved her marriage, and she pushed me to keep trying. She said she too felt trapped as soon as she and the groom exchanged vows. We always hear about men feeling trapped in relationships, but my boss said that many women feel the same way even though our culture discourages us from acknowledging or talking about it."

Linda got Brian into counseling, but it lasted only three visits and ended with both of them disappointed. Linda was finally clear that her feelings were real, but she was still afraid to utter the word "divorce," because she was ashamed to admit that the marriage didn't work. She turned to Roger, a coworker who had been flirting with her for two years. She started a hot and heavy affair with him, eventually giving her the courage to serve Brian with divorce papers. Roger and Linda stayed together for a while, but the flame of passion wore off quickly and they went their separate ways.

Linda's lesson was that relationships founded on sex and convenience, without a serious and committed emotional connection and solid ongoing communication, just don't work out in the long run. When people are young and time is on their side, couples like Linda and Brian, Monica and Max, or Rebecca and Derek often rush into marriage because it seems like the next logical step to take, the right box to check off on life's mandatory checklist. In order to stay together, couples need to understand that marriage is about more than just sex, or a wedding band, or material trappings. And it's never easy. In our culture, too many people see a first marriage as a "loss leader" and find it simpler to walk out rather than doing the real work. The catch is, they never learn the lesson of what it takes to create and maintain a real relationship. They'll carry their same problems and issues with them into the next relationship and on and on. It takes two people to make a marriage last, and unless you put a lot of work into understanding your individual role in the outcome and your contribution to the failure, you're likely to repeat the same pattern with the next person you believe to be your soul mate.

Felicity is a bubbly blonde who was 29 when she came to me for help with a thyroid imbalance. Newly divorced for the second time, she was still shaken by her experience with Albert.

"We met at a party. Albert was bartending, and we struck up a conversation. He asked me if I was single, and when I said yes, he wanted us to meet after he was done with work. I did and we spent the rest of the night talking. Eventually, we wound up in bed at my apartment. Sex was great; we both were tremendously turned on. We started seeing a lot of each other, and every time we would have sex. Our love life was magical, and he was so interesting and smart. He also was very attentive and noticed everything about me, making me feel really great. A short time later, he moved in with me. Everything was moving so smoothly and so wonderfully, I felt I had found my real soul mate.

"Albert was from Europe, and I thought that was another reason why he was so special. I've always heard European men are great lovers and know how to treat their women well. As things progressed, we got engaged and then married. His family did not come to the wedding, but he said it was because they could not afford the expense of the trip. While some of my family and friends thought this was strange, I told him I understood. Marriage was wonderful at first. We had so much fun and laughed all the time. Soon after, I was ready to start thinking of having kids and shared my thoughts with Albert. He was totally on board. However, something did change. One day, a few months later, Albert casually mentioned he had decided to go back home for a while. I assumed I'd go with him, of course, wanting to see his homeland and meet his family at long last. But all he would say was that he had a flight to make that very evening. As he packed a small duffel bag, I began to get a strange feeling in the pit of my stomach. He wouldn't admit it, but I was terrified that he was leaving for good.

"Albert left our beautiful apartment with a small bag and the clothes on his back. There was nothing I could say to stop him. I was in shock and kept telling myself he'd come right back. Instead he cut off all contact with me as soon as he walked out the door. He literally told me he wanted a divorce via text. I never understood why things changed, or what I did wrong. It's been three years now, and I never heard from him again.

"Now I'm not even 30, divorced for the second time, and alone again. My first marriage ended when my husband cheated on me, but we were both very young and right out of college. He cheated on me with one of my girlfriends and then lied about it. I just walked away and never spoke to him again. I never looked at that failure too closely, because I was so young and inexperienced. I've been in therapy for a while now, but I still haven't figured out why I was blindsided twice. I feel like there's something wrong with me that drives men away, but I don't know what it is. Before, I used to go from one relationship to the next, but my therapist has taught me to take a break and figure out who I am and what my wants and needs are before I jump into something new. She also taught me that I'll never learn much about myself while I'm in a relationship, so I need to learn to be alone for a while. I wish my mom had taught me that when I was a kid."

Felicity went from one poor relationship decision to the next, without figuring out what went wrong. She never looked at herself for any of the answers. It may be she's carrying baggage from her childhood she isn't even aware of; maybe she's commitment-phobic, or it may just be that she's insecure and jumps into relationships too fast without making sure there's a real connection there. Whatever Felicity's issues, the culture we live in today places a low value on true commitment and doesn't encourage us to take responsibility for our actions. The media bombards us with news about celebrity divorces, high-profile sexual betrayals, and multiple hookups, sending the inescapable message that people are interchangeable.

YOUNG AND SINGLE WITH KIDS

When the loss of a spouse occurs with young children in the picture, young women and men have a lot more to address. Tall, elegant Sarah, now in her mid-40s, has been a patient of mine for over a decade, and she has shared with me her amazing life journey.

"Jim and I met at a political rally when I was 23 and he was 24. We quickly discovered that we shared a lot more than political views. Chemistry drew us together instantly, and we soon found ourselves talking politics in bed, debating how to save the world together between hot and heavy lovemaking sessions. We both felt we had everything in common and quickly found ourselves deeply in love. After two years, we married and had our two little girls a year and a half apart. We were even trying for another baby. Our life together was great. Even with the children, we made time for the two of us. Sex was always great, because I had a high libido back then and took the lead and Jim was all for it. It was fun; our sex life was fulfilling—complete with sex toys, lingerie, role-playing, and crazy outfits. Jim even told me when the guys at his job talked about wild vacations in Las Vegas or going to strip joints, he just smiled to himself because he had all the excitement he ever wanted and needed at home. I was proud and certainly satisfied.

"One Sunday morning, Jim went to buy milk. The girls always looked forward to his Sunday pancakes with faces made out of banana slices and chocolate syrup. On the way, a bus lost control and totaled Jim's car. The policeman who came to my door told me he died on impact.

"There I was, still in my 20s, a widow with two toddlers. It was more than shocking. I can't even describe how I felt. My life stopped dead at that moment. My sister and her husband moved in with us to help me take care of the girls. I was useless as a mother. I went to therapists, took antidepressants, and went to a few support groups, but no matter what I did, I couldn't find peace.

"Finally, a year later, I went back to work, my sister and her husband went home, and life fell into a new normal routine. Everyone I knew pushed me to go out and meet another man. I can't tell you how many times some well-meaning friend or relative would say to me, 'Sarah, your girls deserve a father.' To me, the girls already had a father, and he was gone. No one could ever replace him. Plus, I had my hands more than full with work and raising the girls as a single mother—there was no room for anyone else.

"But in time, I was so lonely I gave in. I went online and joined a couple of dating sites for widowers. I certainly was popular; I was swamped with inquiries from men ages 25 to 75. I was more overwhelmed and scared than pleased. Who was I supposed to trust? I felt too vulnerable and not sure I even wanted to try it. I'd heard horror stories of men lying and cheating on their wives, just to have sex. The internet seemed like a minefield to me. Plus, the last thing I thought about was sex. The idea of having sex with a new man was still repulsive to me.

"I was tortured by my fear and indecision. But the more I thought about it, the less interested I was in following someone else's idea of what my life should be. I realized that my priority should be raising my girls and providing the best possible life for them. So I did what was right for me and put the entire dating thing on hold. I focused on work and became an executive with a Fortune 100 company, and put both my daughters through Ivy League schools. Then, when I was in my early 40s, I met Larry, who was divorced and 10 years older than me. Our relationship grew out of friendship; sex wasn't what led me to him. We became friends and then sex happened naturally after a few months. Larry and I never married and don't plan to, but we are a real couple. We do everything together, and my daughters love him. Larry is a great man with whom I have lots in common, including great sex. Jim will always be the love of my life—and Larry knows that. He understands it and so do I. After some painful, rocky years, I now believe myself to be very lucky. I know I made the right decisions for me and my girls. Life is good, and I know what a good and solid relationship is all about."

DIVIDED FAMILIES

When marriages with kids end in divorce, the issue of custody rears its ugly head. Unlike their childless counterparts who can just walk away from a failed marriage, divorced parents invariably must remain connected, for the sake of the children. Often, this isn't an easy feat.

Jennifer was married to Josh for 10 years. They wed right out of medical school and both entered exciting careers—she as an anesthesiologist, he as an orthopedic surgeon. They hit life's treadmill running and soon had two children on top of their demanding practices. But as the years passed and their lives grew even busier—as they worked different hours in different hospitals, making different friends—their relationship began to suffer. Life in hospitals is high-pressured and intense; temptation lies around every corner. Eventually, both Jennifer and Josh started seeing other people, and before they even got a chance to examine what had happened to their marriage, it was over.

When they got divorced, neither had a bad thing to say about the other. Jennifer summarized it best. "We just outgrew each other," she said. "Nothing bad, just time took its toll and our marriage couldn't withstand the changes." Neither had regrets nor felt sorry about the divorce. They just decided to move on.

It wasn't so easy for their two daughters, Zoe, age 8, and Sarah, 6. They'd grown up used to having a nanny care for them while their parents worked long hours at the hospitals, but now things changed even more. Since Jennifer and Josh felt shared custody was in the best interest of the girls, they moved close to each other so their daughters could spend half the time which each parent.

Jennifer and Josh both meant well, and on paper, the shared arrangement looked good. At first it seemed to work—until both parents started seriously dating other people who placed new demands on their time and attention. Soon, the girls were spending more time with the housekeepers and nannies than with either parent. The trouble began to manifest itself at school and in the girls' social lives, but due to their busy schedules, neither mother nor father saw the warning signs. By the time they noticed and tried to get their daughters into therapy, the situation was a runaway train. What the girls really needed was consistent parental presence in their lives and a level of supervision and support neither parent was able to provide.

Today, the girls are in their teens and both in boarding schools. Zoe, who suffered more than Sarah, has an eating disorder—a symptom of trying to control her body since as a child she had none. Sarah is very popular, and her life revolves around her school friends. Neither has any interest in going home for the holidays or spending more than the minimum required time with the parents they both feel abandoned them.

Children like Sarah and Zoe are innocent casualties of actions by adults who didn't think about the consequences of their actions. While Josh and Jennifer felt their divorce was inconsequential, it changed their little daughters' lives. I'm not saying it was the divorce alone that caused the problems for the children, but I do believe that at least one committed and present parent figure willing to put the kids before his or her own needs might have changed the outcome of this all-too-common story.

LEARNING FROM ALONE TIME

In our society, single women often tend to find it more difficult than men to find new partners. In fact, they fare better when they spend time alone, examining their choices and seeking to understand the reasons their relationships didn't work out so they might be able to prevent the same mistake from leaving them unhappy again. While being suddenly single may be traumatic, at the end of the day, it can offer both women and men another chance to gain more insight and perspective on their lives opening the door for better choices.

As I've tried to explain throughout the previous chapters, I believe indiscriminate sex with multiple partners is both physically and emotionally risky regardless of what some women might want to believe.

Many of the gay male patients I work with lament the inconsequential way sex is treated in the gay culture. My patient Mark, a 36-year-old attractive gay man, complains bitterly that it is almost impossible to find a man willing to get involved in a long-term relationship when sex is so freely available in the gay-male community. Mark envies heterosexual couples, because he believes the culture is about commitment and long-term relationships. I don't want to disappoint him, but the truth is, heterosexual and gay or lesbian relationships are similar in a lot of ways. The cultures may present different perspectives, yet the underlying truth is invariably the same: a couple trying to turn the initial sexually motivated relationship into a long-term sexually and emotionally stable lifestyle.

There are many women in their late 30s and early 40s who find themselves single with diminishing prospects for finding truly desirable partners. This is a big problem, and complaints in this age group only grow more numerous. Single women who want to have sex cannot seem to find the right partner to have sex with. The only available men appear to be married, decades younger, bad boys, or old and boring.

When the right guy is nowhere in sight is a good time to spend time alone figuring out your own personal truth and how your expectations fit into the reality of your own life. Denial and outdoing the guys with ever-increasing numbers of sex partners won't help you feel better. At the end of the day, looking at your life honestly and keeping your expectations honest will lead to a more fulfilling and healthier life.

But just because you're now alone doesn't mean you have to deny or submerge your sexuality. If you are single and your sex drive is high, masturbation is a safe and healthy way to continue enjoying sexual release while you're in between relationships or waiting for "the right one" to come along, or even if you're in a relationship that no longer provides sufficient sexual satisfaction. As a doctor, I have always been baffled by taboos against masturbation, because it is a natural biological function that crosses all cultures, ages, sexes, and geographical boundaries.

Men are raised to feel free and even encouraged to masturbate. Everywhere we turn, male masturbation is playfully acknowledged as a normal thing in our society. It may seem like a hard pill to swallow, but studies have shown that married men masturbate even more than single ones. Even Alfred Kinsey found that 40 percent of men and 30 percent of women in relationships still masturbate, and that was decades ago. More recent surveys in *Playboy* and *Redbook* place the figures at 72 percent and 68 percent, respectively.[4]

Interestingly, no studies have found that men have a greater biological need than women to masturbate. However, cultural attitudes toward female masturbation have been more negative and discouraging. When I talk to my female patients about masturbation, even the younger ones sometimes still get embarrassed! Many studies and much psychiatric research aim to help women feel better about and understand their own bodies, to explore them and to learn to relax and feel entitled to please themselves sexually without a partner. There is a myth that masturbation negatively affects self-esteem. For women, the opposite seems to be true—studies have shown that women who masturbate feel better about themselves and are more confident and comfortable with their own bodies.[5] It is a far healthier pastime than seeking the fleeting admiration of a temporary lover, who may cause more harm than good to a woman's self-esteem or confidence—not to mention, may provide little sexual satisfaction and increase the risk of STDs.

Since we are no longer Puritans and live in an almost egalitarian society, encouraging women to explore, understand, and find pleasure in their own bodies is a requirement for evolution. Masturbation can be both a release in a solo activity and part of a couple's healthy sex life. As Woody Allen famously said, "Don't knock masturbation. It's sex with someone I love."

VIBRATORS

While vibrators are the most popular sex toys sold in the U.S., you might want to know their checkered history and start looking at them as a little more than just sex toys.

In the 19th century, before it was known that women had orgasms or could enjoy sex, our esteemed medical establishment labeled sexually dissatisfied women as suffering from "hysteria." In the 1880s an English doctor, Joseph Mortimer Granville, developed the first vibrator and also brought into question the entire diagnosis of hysteria.

Vibrators entered the medical therapeutics world as well as that of beauty. But while we all know vibrators are fun sex toys, we don't all realize they can be important in providing sexual satisfaction and orgasms and improving women's pleasure in sex.

Vibrators may appear to be part and parcel of the sexual awakening of women and the newest sex toy party trick, but, in fact, they are legitimate and medically sound devices that help improve hormone balance and sexual gratification at all ages.

Just watch the 2011 movie *Hysteria* and you will see how far we've come and realize now how much further we still must go.

SOLUTIONS FOR THE SINGLE WOMAN

When you are young and find yourself without a romantic partner:

- Take the time to heal, to get to know yourself and become the best version of yourself, a person you like and are proud to be.
- Be honest with yourself and look at your actions rather than at what your partner did wrong to cause the breakup.
- Find a reliable support system of people who can understand what you're going through and have had similar experiences.
- If you got divorced, take a hard look at the marriage and come clean about why things didn't work out. Take responsibility and commit to becoming a better person and better partner for the next time.

- Before you get into a new relationship, spend some time with a good therapist or coach (life or dating) to understand what you really want and need and why things went awry, so you don't repeat harmful patterns.
- Spend time alone. Then take a hard look at yourself to figure out if marriage is really the right lifestyle for you.
- Don't judge yourself too harshly. Learn your lesson and move on. It's all part of your journey.
- Know that marriage is about two people, and you don't have control over the other person's actions.
- Learn what's best for you. You're not being selfish. You're becoming an adult.
- Follow your instincts and learn not to ignore your gut. Your gut is always right.

CHAPTER 7

SEX AND PARENTHOOD: AN UNLIKELY COMBINATION

"Parents are the last people on earth
who ought to have children."

—Samuel Butler

Whenever I hear a married woman in her late 30s or 40s say her sex life is fabulous and very frequent, that she and her husband can't keep their hands off each other, I know one of three things is going on: It's a new marriage, there are no children in the household, or…she is lying. I know from my own and my patients' experience that when kids are taking up your time and energy—mental and emotional as well as physical—it's just about impossible to enjoy sex as freely as you used to when it was just you and your partner. Those stories of unbridled sex anytime, anywhere are reserved for the very young and definitely for those who are very free of responsibility. Once children enter the picture, it's officially autumn in the sexual life cycle.

Remember those carefree weekends when the two of you would sleep late, letting the hours drift by without getting out of bed? Can you recall the days with your new love when sex was passionate, lustful, and totally spontaneous? How about those candlelit anniversary, birthday, or everyday romantic dinners, just the two of you, without friends or family to entertain? Didn't they invariably lead to great lovemaking? When you are at the beginning of a romantic sexual relationship, you can't imagine that your relationship won't always be like that—hot sex and intensely intimate moments, just the two of you. You are the center of your universe, and nothing the outside world can throw at you will ever change that. Remember?

All that changes when a baby arrives.

TRYING TO CONCEIVE

In most couples planning to start a family, the woman finds herself pregnant before any actual effort has gotten underway. They are the lucky ones. When two people make the conscious decision to have children, the whole mood of their sexuality changes. Even if getting pregnant doesn't take much effort, it still changes the goal of sex from lovemaking for enjoyment, an expression of love and pleasure, to the job of completing our biological mission. For many couples, this dramatically changes everything about sex and intimacy in their marriage.

Just think of those women who don't have an easy time getting pregnant. Those who struggle to conceive, where monthly ovulation becomes the time when they *must* have sex. How sexy is that? My male patients and female patients' husbands faced with this situation consistently tell me they lose interest in sex with their spouses because they suddenly feel used. They no longer feel like virile men who are wanted and desired by their partners, but rather like utilitarian sperm donors, simply useful baby-making machines. No man wants to feel like that.

Then come the months of stress and anguish, when the pee stick fails to show a positive sign, the dreaded period arrives right on time, and becoming pregnant turns into an obsession. Not only can this dim the passion of a previously active and passionate sex life, but it can also ruffle the edges or even destroy the entire relationship.

How does this happen? Since hormones are my specialty—and hormones are crucial determinants when trying to conceive—I spend a lot of time talking with patients, friends, and acquaintances about what's really going on behind the bedroom doors during this time. Again and again, I've seen previously relaxed, practical women turn every ounce of their attention and energy exclusively to getting pregnant, regardless of whether they are successful career women or homemakers. On the other hand, the woman's partner continues to interact with and exist in the outside world. Even when men also desire children, they don't narrow their focus to the point that getting pregnant is the only thing that matters in their lives. They can switch gears and focus on work, watch a football game, hang out with their buddies, and continue living as they did before the onset of the "we must get pregnant now" phase of the relationship.

Because it's her body at the center of the conception goal, the woman often finds herself becoming obsessed. Every period is a minor tragedy, a disappointment; every friend who is pregnant, a reminder of her own failure. Wherever she turns, in every aspect of her life—every magazine article, TV show, or movie, or baby passed on the street—many a woman trying to get pregnant sees reminders of what she so desperately wants. Too often this baby-making single-mindedness becomes the rule rather than a rare exception as the period comes and pregnancy doesn't immediately occur.

With every passing month that pregnancy doesn't happen, sex increasingly becomes just a means to an end. How does something that was so joyous and exciting a moment ago turn into an anxiety-filled chore? When I ask a large number of couples in the throes of trying to conceive I hear a similar story.

In their early 30s, Georgia and Tom were married for almost three years. They took the time to build a strong relationship during their courtship, loved each other passionately, and enjoyed frequent, passionate sex. Both had highly successful jobs they loved and enjoyed the finer things in life. As a couple, they were the envy of their friends. As they watched all those friends begin to have children, Georgia and Tom decided it was time for them to start as well. Georgia went off the birth control pills she had been on for almost 10 years, and they decided to let nature take its course.

The first three months, they had sex the usual way, whenever it struck them, which was morning, noon, and night. They were both young and healthy and figured it wouldn't take long. They told themselves that getting pregnant meant more sex, which made them even happier.

But Georgia didn't get pregnant. After three months, she started buying ovulation predictor sticks in bulk, to make sure she knew exactly when her ovulation would take place. Once the stick turned positive, she knew they had a 24- to 48-hour window to get pregnant. Georgia began demanding that Tom immediately join her in the bedroom to perform. The quality and quantity of sex changed. Tom felt they were no longer intimate. It seemed like Georgia wanted only to get his sperm. Georgia admitted this was true, but she saw it as a good thing. Didn't they often, in the heat of passion, whisper to one another, "I want to have your baby"? Wouldn't this be the culmination of those moments?

After another few months of regular periods, Georgia went to the gynecologist to make sure she didn't have any physical abnormalities. She was relieved to learn that she was healthy. And yet, as the months passed, her periods continued to arrive like clockwork. This sent the previously happily married pair to a couples therapist, since they were no longer getting along the way they used to. Sex had become a chore, and communication between them was breaking down fast. Tom seemed keener on being with his buddies or working late then hanging out with Georgia, which used to be his favorite pastime. The therapist helped Tom admit how hurt and left out he felt, now that Georgia seemed to care more about getting pregnant than about Tom or his feelings. Although he too wanted children very much, he felt the process of trying to conceive was destroying their relationship.

But Georgia didn't get the message. Caught up in pregnancy fever, she began to harp on Tom, haranguing him about his disinterest in the process and accusing him of not caring about having a family as much as he'd led her to believe. In time, Tom had his sperm evaluated, and it too was normal. The couple went to a fertility clinic and underwent a couple of in-utero insemination (IUI) treatments that didn't do much, leading finally to IVF, which finally left Georgia pregnant but Tom resentful of everything it took to get there.

Eventually they welcomed a healthy baby girl into the world. Tom thought at last their relationship would now return to normal. Instead, Georgia became even more obsessed—this time, with her new baby daughter. She hired a baby nurse, whom she never let near the baby. She took off three months from work to tend to the newborn. Tom appreciated her devotion, but inside he felt even more alienated. When they visited my office when the baby was six months old, Tom confessed he felt the family structure had changed. It was now Georgia and the baby, and Tom was like a lonely moon orbiting their cozy little planet. The road back to creating one family, to integrating the two partners into the new life, was already paved with resentment. For this formerly blissful couple, the baby they had prayed for had become a stumbling block to their intimacy and sexuality. They wouldn't have sex for another year, as Georgia doted on the baby and Tom struggled to accept his new status as an outsider.

And Tom was not alone. A large number of new parents describe the year after they welcome their first child as the most difficult and trying for the marriage. Expectations change, the relationship changes, and the parents have to seriously readjust in order to make it to the next level of the relationship as a team rather than as two separate individuals.

PREGNANCY, CHILDREN, AND A NEW WORLD OF SEX

A lot of men talk about being afraid to have sex with their pregnant wives because they don't want to injure the baby. Why doesn't anyone tell them there's no need to worry? There's a uterus (a very thick muscle) and lots of water (amniotic fluid) protecting the fetus from their penis! The fetus is *totally safe*.

In many cases women say their sex drive rises significantly during pregnancy, and their mates describe sex as being rich and plentiful during these pregnancies. With some other pregnancies, women lose their sex drive altogether and couples cling to the threads of sexuality with more holding and cuddling than actual sex. It all depends on hormone levels and environmental factors, as well as the individual genetics and personalities involved.

The most shocking thing I've found—from patients and own experience—is that so many women are blindsided by what happens to their sex life after the baby is born. If women are unprepared for the transition from being young and carefree to being married and trying to get pregnant, they are even less prepared for what happens after they have children.

When women go to their obstetricians for their six-week postpartum follow-up, they're usually told they're fine and can resume normal sexual activity. Really? Most of my patients come crying to me about how they feel abandoned by their doctors, who send them off back to having sex so casually, not taking into consideration the changes in their bodies or emotions since they gave birth. If the woman delivered vaginally, which most do, the pain of intercourse the first time after the delivery is often worse than the pain of losing one's virginity. And how sexy does a woman feel after she has just delivered a baby and her belly is floating above the waterline in the tub while she is taking a bath?

And what about the man? Most men are next to their partners in the delivery room. While this is a highly charged emotional moment, some men are still shocked to realize that they and the baby share the same vagina. After birth, their desire for sex may be dimmed by their reluctance to hurt the mother of their child. Suddenly, the wife is now the mother of their child, not their personal sex toy anymore. It's a difficult reality for many men to accept.

Here's the naked truth: Sex after having a baby is not the same as sex before pregnancy. In many marriages, this is a transformative event. Sex is no longer about passion or lust. Instead, it is about making children, following the rules of our culture that state we must continue to have sex with the husband or wife we no longer view the same way we did before the baby was born. And there is no warning information nor instruction manual to go along with this dramatic change to help us cope and adjust to the new paradigm.

Jean, a 35-year-old patient, told me that while she was in labor with her firstborn, she realized her husband would be seeing the baby come out of her vagina and she thought that might turn him off permanently to sex with her. So she asked her husband to stand by her head and hold her hand while she delivered. This way he never really saw their daughter being delivered. She also made sure that at the six-week mark, she and her husband started having sex again in spite of the pain. Now, three years later, she swears those two actions kept her marriage vibrant and their sex life strong.

Jean and her husband are among the lucky ones. They have a strong marriage and Jean's focus has stayed with the marriage. She loves their daughter to pieces, but she says the marriage comes first. She learned from her mother what to expect and how to behave in the marriage after having a baby; her mother, Jean told me, still has a great marriage to her father after 40 years and three children.

Too many people don't take into account the upheaval caused by bringing a new human being into what used to be a two-person relationship. You can't leave the baby at the hospital. All this little being knows how to do is cry when hungry, tired, or needing a diaper change. The baby doesn't care what the parents want. This is the time when you and your spouse must decide whether the baby will become an addition to your life, or you will become a slave to your baby. Whichever decision you make will significantly affect your marriage.

You're both also facing the challenge of parenting. If you're the father, what will your involvement in the process be? If you're the mother, most likely you will have to learn to manage your expectations about your husband's involvement with the newborn. Staying up all night, breastfeeding and pumping milk from your engorged breasts will become the new norm. For some men, this is scary and confusing, and at the very least, it's not the sexiest way to see a wife. Most women today expect their partners to be present and take an active role in the life of the little creature in the crib. All these issues and more must be discussed and clarified by the two of you, because they will certainly affect your marriage and your sex life.

Sleepless nights, weight that seems to get stuck and refuses to drop back to prepregnancy levels, and physical and emotional exhaustion define a woman's first year of the new baby's life, while the couple transforms into a family. To keep it together, you have to remember that the *two of you* are the nucleus of this family. If you make time to talk and grab alone time, while trying to hold on to as much as you can of your prebaby sexuality, you will weather the storm and come out on the other side a family and a happy couple. If not, your marriage might get lost in the deluge.

NOW THERE ARE BABIES

After the first couple of years with a child in the house, you may think that once the little one goes to nursery school, your sex life will return to normal. Sorry to say, that's unlikely to happen. Babies that become children are the start of a 20-year phase that will change everything you thought you knew about your marriage. Small children, tweens, teens, and beyond: As long as children live with you and even after they leave the home, they're going to put significant limits on your sex life unless you and your spouse are both determined to prevent that from happening. Damage control is totally possible—if you are truly committed to protecting your sex life as a significant part of your marriage and to manifesting your love for one another by keeping sexuality an integral part of your life.

Maybe you are a stay-at-home mom who spends hours with your children. You prepare breakfast, pack lunches and drive the kids to school. Maybe in the afternoon you take them to after-school activities. In between, you clean and shop, work part-time, or volunteer for various school events. Your days are filled with demanding childcentric duties, and you rarely make time for yourself and even less for your partner. Vacations, which you and your husband used to think of as romantic stress-relieving getaways, are now all about going wherever the kids can be happy and entertained. On those rare occasions when grandparents babysit for a weekend, you are still under pressure. Instead of enjoying a relaxing time together, you wonder what is going on at home. As for your husband, he tries to show you he still desires you sexually, though maybe he's not as demonstrative as he was before the kids arrived. You need attention too but can't switch off from mommy mode to sexual siren at a moment's notice, and that dichotomy affects your sexual interactions. Worrying about the kids and everything about them takes precedence. This is a time when many couples struggle. How they manage this transition often determines the outcome of the marriage. Protecting and keeping your sex life alive and well involves attention, honesty, understanding, communication, and lots of work.

Maura came from a large, close-knit family. She met her husband, Liam, at a family affair when she was 16. They got married when they were both 20, welcomed their first child at 21, the second two years later, the third after three years, and the fourth 18 months after that. The kids were healthy and lively, and grandparents on both sides helped out. Since they all lived close to each other, babysitting wasn't a problem.

Maura and Liam lived in a colonial house with a white picket fence; Liam made a good living at his father-in-law's construction company, and Maura took care of the home and kids. She was also very active in the community church and the kids' school. She gardened and made cookies—her baking quickly became famous throughout the neighborhood. By the time Maura and Liam found themselves in their late 20s, they had already achieved the American dream. But there was a growing emptiness underneath the perfect surface.

Maura and Liam had moved through different phases of life at such high speed, they lost the very essence of what had brought them together. At the beginning of their relationship, they were getting the sex and intimacy parts right. Their children were conceived out of love and devotion, and Maura and Liam shared the same vision for their life plan. A decade later, their sexual connection had become an obligation. Maura no longer felt that Liam appreciated her. When they had first gotten together, he used to constantly tell her she was beautiful, and in bed he paid special loving attention to every part of her body. Those days were long gone. Now she felt taken for granted. Once in a while, in the middle of the night or in the wee hours of the morning, Liam would turn over in bed and just enter her without warning or foreplay. If she pushed him away, he'd just grunt and go back to sleep. If she ever wanted to talk about it in the morning, he never seemed to remember what had happened. Maura was increasingly lonely and frustrated.

When Maura came to see me, she told me she needed hormones because she had no sex drive. She hadn't had an orgasm in over five years—pretty much coinciding with when their last child was conceived. Liam was uncomfortable talking about sex and stonewalled her on the subject. When Maura went to her mother and sisters with the complaint, she was shocked to hear them tell her there was nothing wrong with Liam. Her mom, married to her dad for over 40 years, told her that no married couples with young children had great sex, if they had any sex at all. This was the rule rather than the exception, she said, and it didn't mean there was a problem with the marriage.

"I can't believe I'm only 28 and I feel like my mom at 60. Am I doomed to feel unappreciated and sexless for the rest of my life?" Maura asked me.

I was able to balance her hormones, gave her a little progesterone before her period and testosterone during the entire cycle, and she started to feel better physically. I also recommended she see a therapist, and after a few sessions, she started going to the gym, lost weight, and became more interested in her appearance. Liam immediately noticed Maura's new look—thinner, more vibrant, new haircut, new style—and seemed to wake up a bit. Within a few weeks, they took their first vacation alone in years. And so a new chapter in their married life started, one marked by paying more attention to each other's needs. They loved each other and realized that a marriage works only with the original couple, not the children, at its center. As the kids started to make their own way, Maura and Liam enjoyed their time together more and realized how important they were to one another, leading to a great connected and healthy marriage.

This story is not rare, but the outcome differs for individual couples. Those who do the hard work of keeping the couple at the heart of the relationship from which all other relationships flow usually forge solid and lasting marriages. Those who let the children be the primary focus, using the children and work to avoid intimacy, not doing the work to keep the marriage together, often end up divorced or in less savory arrangements—having affairs, lying, becoming isolated, and living in a cold-war environment rather than building solid and enduring marriages.

WHEN CHILDREN RUN THE SHOW

Sometimes women are so overwhelmed by the responsibilities of raising children they preemptively put a halt on their sexuality.

"I never thought I would repeat my parents' history," said Nina, a 37-year-old mother of a two-and-a-half-year-old. "Until I was seven, I slept in the same room with them. They both doted on me but barely spoke to each other, and have a chilly marriage to this day. When I got pregnant with Ethan, I swore to myself and to Joel that we would never be the coddling parents who let their kids ruin their marriage. But after Ethan was born, something changed in me. I became obsessed. All I could see and hear was Ethan. Joel disappeared from my radar screen. I immediately moved the port-a crib into the bedroom, saying it would be easier to hear and feed him that way. Joel didn't like it, but what could he do? He rationalized it as a phase that would pass. Months after I delivered, Joel tried to have sex with me. I felt uncomfortable and didn't want him touching my breasts—it was like now they belonged to Ethan. Things went from bad to worse, and our sex life dried up completely. Joel seemed tolerant of all the excuses, but I knew something had to be done.

"I know Joel still loves me and has been patient, but he often locks the bathroom door and he takes long showers. I know he's masturbating. When I try to talk to him about it, he denies it and changes the subject. Since I have no sex drive now, I guess it's the only thing he can do without getting the marriage into serious trouble. But I know at our age and stage in life, my husband masturbating and me having no sex drive are a prescription for disaster for the marriage in the long run."

REPERCUSSIONS OF MISCARRIAGE

"I went through a lot to get our twins," said Jessica, a first-time mom at 42. "I got pregnant five times, but I always had a miscarriage. They were not only emotionally traumatic but big stressors to my body. By my late 30s I had given up on the idea that I could have my own children. My husband is the most supportive man I know, and we both wanted to become parents, so we decided to adopt. No one prepared us for the process. It dragged on forever and caused us a slew of disappointments and rejections. Ultimately, we got lucky. When we finally saw our adopted twin girls, I knew instantly I was in love. I couldn't love them more if I'd carried them myself. They've brought more happiness into our lives than I could have ever imagined possible.

"The problem is, after all the miscarriages, I've come to associate sexual intercourse with failure. Needless to say, my sex drive is practically nonexistent. I don't want to lose my husband, especially now that we've built such a beautiful family. But I can't seem to lift myself out of this deep hole. It's sad: I'm so happy to be a mother, but I don't believe I can be a lover anymore. I've talked to other women like me and read similar stories on the internet. Every woman says the same thing. Once you associate sex with failure, you just turn off. I hope it's not permanent, and I hope that if I keep talking it through with my husband, I'll eventually make it out of this phase."

THE HORMONE EFFECT

During pregnancy, myriad hormones help the female body support the development and growth of the fetus in the womb. These hormones are estrogen, progesterone, testosterone, human chorionic gonadotropic hormone (hCG), and many others. In the brain, they stimulate the production of what we know as "feel good" hormones, like serotonin and dopamine, which keep pregnant women in a great mood (once they get into the second trimester and are no longer nauseated and exhausted) that we commonly refer to as "glowing."

As the baby is born, the pituitary gland releases another hormone—oxytocin—which facilitates an immediate bond between mother and baby. I mentioned it in previous chapters, but after birth it has another role. With the help of oxytocin, lactation begins and the uterus starts to shrink back to its original size, which is about as small as a hazelnut. The other pregnancy hormones precipitously drop, because they are no longer needed to keep the baby alive and growing inside the mother's womb. As this magical process unfolds, a woman also loses the many hormones made by another organ, the placenta, which exists solely to feed and support the growth of the fetus during pregnancy. All these losses and sudden hormone fluctuations lead to tremendous shifts in the new mother's body and mood.

As the new baby is brought to the mother's breast to start suckling, to make skin-to-skin contact, the release of the bonding hormone oxytocin leads to a miraculous transformation. Men standing by often observe that their wives go into a trancelike state as they hold and gaze at their new babies. And while men also make oxytocin and bond with both baby and mother, they don't produce it in the same quantities women do. Because of biology and culture, men and women bond differently with their new babies.

A woman has to adjust to a significantly different and often permanent new physical and emotional identity after 40 weeks of pregnancy. Many women never return to the people they were before. Over the 40 weeks of pregnancy, women transition from being wives and lovers to mothers. The entire focus of the family structure shifts, and many men complain that they lose both their marriages and their sex lives with their wives the moment their babies are born. This is not an exaggeration. It's a hormonal and cultural fact of life.

The question is, will this situation destroy the marriage, or will it lead to a deeper, more adult phase of life that may still be full of passion but also more profound and satisfying? The answer lies somewhere among anatomy, biology, and culture, with the two married people trying to define their relationship to one another and the position of the children in their lives. All these issues are fluid and ever-changing, making it often difficult for couples to navigate their relationships.

WOMEN VERSUS MEN HORMONES

As women enter their late 30s to mid-40s, the hormone balance starts to shift again. Ovulation may no longer occur like clockwork, and estrogen and progesterone ratios change from the predictable fluctuations of the 20s. Testosterone, the most abundant hormone in women as well as men, may also start to get out of balance. As a result, physical and emotional symptoms appear. Loss of libido is one of many changes women experience. Hot flashes, mood swings, irritability, night sweats, and emotional volatility before periods make life even more complicated when women are raising kids, tending to the family, and going to work. Sexuality moves to the back burner, and more women "fake it" than we will ever know.

Change is on the horizon for men as well, but it starts later. Testosterone is the hormone stereotypically associated with what we view as manliness—with muscle-building ability and aggression and, most of all, a strong and omnipresent sex drive. The truth is that men also make estrogen, and it's the *balance* of estrogen and testosterone that determines their well-being. As men age, their testosterone levels drop and their sex drive flags, along with their energy and motivation at work and home. More men experience issues than we hear about, because our male-dominated culture still isn't comfortable discussing them in the open. Male menopause, or andropause, is now in the same place menopause was for women two decades ago. Rarely talked about yet another normal phase of life experienced by all with its own uncomfortable symptoms and life-altering outcomes.

Ironically, we're in the midst of an infertility epidemic in men. Low sperm counts are on the rise, linked to various environmental factors ranging from too-frequent bicycle riding to exposure to industrial chemicals and heavy metals. Lifestyle choices may also be contributing factors. These include tobacco, drug, and alcohol use and the obesity pandemic. What a man does for a living also matters. Sitting too long at a computer, sedentary lifestyles, and high stress may also lower sperm count. Use of anabolic steroids to build muscles leads to testicular atrophy and low sperm counts as well.[1] Very little news of this pervasive issue reaches the general public. Slowly, though, the word is getting out, and solutions have to follow.

THE MALE PERSPECTIVE

From the moment a man gets engaged to be married, his sex life changes drastically. Men, who biologically have a longer reproductive lifespan than women, are also culturally indoctrinated to believe there is little rush to commit to having a family or kids. Men are also encouraged by society to keep their focus more outside the home and family than women are.

Our culture expects men to be providers, to be interested in sports and math and to feel free to explore life with looser boundaries than women. Nonetheless, many men are also very sensitive, and little is written about that. (I recommend the book by Abraham Morgentaler mentioned previously, *Why Men*

Fake It.) Men, like women, seek validation and love. They also need a tremendous amount of reinforcement and recognition, and when the woman they love stops noticing them in favor of the child they created together, their disappointment is palpable. Since most men are primary nurturers less frequently than women, society pays a lot less attention to their emotional needs and expects less of their involvement with babies.

In our society and in relationships as well as biologically, men and women bring different strengths and weaknesses to the table. When they serve to complement one another, these differences help them raise healthy children, have good relationships, and contribute to a well-balanced society.

The sexual revolution of the 1960s raised awareness about the discrimination against women and the daunting barriers of gender inequality, but it also generated a score of other problems that our society is still sorting out. One issue is that many men now feel superfluous, since more women than ever are the main breadwinners in the family, running more than 46 percent of American households. When the wife is the primary wage earner in a marriage, the balance in the relationship changes dramatically. In a 2013 study, the National Bureau of Economic Research concluded that in households where the wife earns more than the husband, the couple is 15 percent less likely to report that the marriage is very happy, 32 percent are more likely to report marital troubles, and 46 percent are more likely to have discussed separation.[2]

This was the subject of *The New York Times* article in 2013.[3] Citing Pew Research Center analysis, it relates how the dynamics of the family have changed. For instance:

- Married women in the workplace are no longer viewed as unusual.

- Single mothers account for more than 25 percent of primary providers.

- By 2012, 32 percent of women reported that they preferred to work full-time over part-time or not working at all. By comparison, in 2007 only 20 percent of women polled felt that way.

- The 2008 recession, which resulted in layoffs that affected men in construction and manufacturing jobs, among others, pushed women into the position of main earner in many families.

- In our strained economy, two paychecks are becoming necessary for most families to live "comfortably."

The shifting cultural role of women has left men in a position where they too have to adjust their expectations and find their new place. Since the focus is turning more to women, less attention has been paid to evaluating the impact of these socioeconomic shifts on men's sexuality and role in the family structure. While men are still free to roam in their youthful, single mode, their roles and the expectations of them change dramatically when they commit to one woman in one relationship. The early phases of family life—trying to conceive, having a pregnant partner, and after a baby is born—are the acute phases of this cataclysmic transition, requiring crucial adjustments. All the factors involved directly affect the course and outcome of marriages far more than we may want to admit.

Once a child enters a home, the sex life of the husband changes yet again. A man who genuinely wanted kids may become conflicted between his love for his new child and his resentment over his disappearing sex life and the dramatic change in his relationship with his wife. Jacob, 32, the father of a one-year-old boy, described a situation at home causing him both pain and confusion.

"I love my son. I love my wife. What I don't love is the lack of physical and emotional closeness between us. I miss sex with Emily, but I also miss the time we shared together before there was a child, when it was only two of us and I didn't feel forced to compete for love and attention with my own son. I feel sad when I remember how much time we had when we were just the two of us. I loved having sex and feeling close to my wife. I knew that my son's birth would change some things, but I didn't imagine everything would shift so drastically. Why has he become the center of Emily's life? Where is my place now? I feel I've been sidelined by a rival. Does this mean I've lost the sex and close-ness with my wife forever? And I also feel guilty about resenting my own son. I wanted him so much, and now I see him as an interloper, an intruder."

Then there is Dan, 37, who explained that, "when Jen and I got married seven years ago, we didn't plan to have children and we made a great life together. When Jen got pregnant, we were stunned: not unhappy—excited but also scared. Jen always said she wasn't really maternal, but as soon as Addie was born, some-thing changed inside her. It's lovely to see that side of Jen, but now I feel left out. I think back to when I was growing up. My dad came home every night for supper, paid the bills and busied himself fixing things around the house. My mom concentrated all her energies on my brother and me. I wonder if my dad felt the same way I do now. I'm not ashamed to admit that I miss the days before we became parents. I feel like having children should come with a warning. Why isn't anyone telling you about it before the kids come?"

Martin, 40, expressed another point of view. "Annie was my dream girl. From the moment I saw her in a bikini on the beach, I knew she was the one for me. Almost a decade has passed since that day. We're both health-conscious, and fitness is part of our daily life. Annie had our first daughter and worked out until the day she delivered. She was back at the gym two weeks after the baby's birth and back to her slim self within a couple of months. But now, 18 months after she gave birth to our second child, she is still trying to lose the extra 30 pounds she gained while she was pregnant. She says that she doesn't feel attractive, that until she is back to 'fighting weight' she won't feel sexy. I'm afraid to tell her that I agree. I want—need—sex, but I'm having a hard time thinking of sex with her. The way she looks now is matronly, and to tell you the truth that is a turn-off. I know I should be more supportive and help her feel better, but I spend more time thinking of other women and watching porn. I actually prefer to masturbate than have sex with her right now. I feel ashamed I'm not a better partner, but this is the truth. I'm sure I'm not the only man who feels that way under similar circumstances."

Rob, 36, told a different story. "We started a family as soon as we got married. We both come from big families, and we planned on having four children. We were lucky to get them quickly and without trouble. We love them; they are pure joy. Penny and I grew up together, and as adults we shared one main goal in life: to be parents. But, to be honest, we didn't get to spend a lot of time alone after we got married. Sex was fine, but it was always squeezed in between commitments to family and friends. There were always members of our families around, with get-togethers and holidays and any excuse for a party. Sometimes we vacationed with her parents, so if we even did it, it was always a quickie in the back of the house, or the bathroom, or somewhere no one would catch us. Not much changed after the kids came, as far as private time is concerned.

"Our lives are super busy and sex, when it happens, is still on the run, but the excitement is totally gone. I enjoy it with Penny, but I feel like it's an obligation rather than an important part of our life as a married couple. In addition to raising the kids, we both work demanding jobs and I take a lot of business trips. Once, a couple of years ago, I met a woman at an industry event, and we ended up having sex. It was amazing; we spent an entire night having sex in a hotel room. For me this was something I had never experienced before. I never planned this; I'm not the kind of guy who's a player. But when I got home, I couldn't get what had happened out of my head. The woman and I kept in touch for a while, and I actually thought about leaving my family, because the experience was so exhilarating and such a change from my sex life with my wife that I wanted more. But the woman was married too, and she ultimately broke it off. I realize that since I did it once, it may happen again. My wife is my best friend and I would never leave her, but I realize now that sex is more important to me than I was willing to admit. I'm torn between my need for sex and my love for my family."

We can't ignore these cases that reflect how profoundly marriages are affected once children enter the picture, but I've found it's something no one wants to talk about. It's a fact that in most marriages—for most men and women—sexuality is important and quite defining, especially when adults are in their prime. Ironically, a recent study indicates that the more egalitarian the marriage in terms of shared chores and responsibilities, the less frequently a couple is likely to have sex.[4] Both men and women report very high degrees of overall happiness in "50–50" marriages, but the numbers show that couples who play out more traditional gender roles in their lives are generally more active in the bedroom. There are few marriages that survive without sex during the reproductive years, so this makes maintaining a sexually active marriage even more of a balancing act when responsibilities are shared 50–50. When highly sexual relationships during the teens, 20s, and even 30s and 40s change overnight into sexless partnerships focused on tending to the children's needs once they come along, the effect is dramatic and can't be ignored without dire consequences. I tell my patients to be prepared for this transition and to make intelligent and thoughtful choices along the way. Most of all, staying honest and communicating—even about the hard stuff—with your partner is your best chance at saving a marriage in transition, maintaining intimacy, and creating an even stronger union.

SOLUTIONS WHEN HAVING A CHILD DISRUPTS YOUR SEX LIFE

§ Be honest and communicate with each other.

§ While trying to conceive, don't let your desire to get pregnant put your relationship on the back burner. Try to remember the two of you came first.

§ Accept the truth that things change, and prepare for this ahead of time by talking things through. Encourage each other and provide loving praise. Notice each other and reinforce the positives.

§ Let go of the notions that the same steamy sex of your teens and 20s must continue and defines a good relationship in your 30s and 40s. Create a new reality, the reality of a great marriage with sex and children in it.

§ Accept that the flush of initial passion does go away, and that doesn't mean you are losing your marriage or must forget about sex in order to have a family and a real relationship.

§ Make sex a priority and take time for yourselves as a couple, regardless of your responsibilities to the rest of the world.

§ Make "date night" a rule in your household and abide by it just like brushing your teeth or any other good habits.

§ Know that sex doesn't always have to be intercourse. It can be sensual and loving caressing and hugging and telling one another how desirable you are. Cuddle and make out and see how wonderful that feels, and how it connects you in times when your mind is not on intercourse.

§ Don't succumb to intentional oversight and denial! It may be painful, but you and your spouse need to talk to each other about what you're going through if things are going to get better and you are going to withstand the changes that having children brings to your relationship.

§ Realize that trading partners rarely works. You will get to the same place with the next "love of your life" even if the sex starts out hot and heavy again.

§ Unless serious damage has been done to your marriage—cheating, lying, deception, loss of love, and lack of communication—you are better off working on what you have than moving on.

CHAPTER 8

WELCOME TO YOUR
EMPTY NEST

*"Middle age is when you're faced with two
temptations and you choose the one that will get you
home by nine o'clock."*

—Ronald Reagan

Congratulations! You've survived the child-rearing years and you're finally seeing the light at the end of the tunnel of parenting as your primary job in life. It's a bittersweet time, filled with laughter, tears, and conflicting feelings of anticipation, relief, and deep sadness. You and your spouse try to keep your emotions in check as you drive your youngest child to the college dorm or to a new apartment. Maybe your child is already living with a partner, engaged, or even married. No matter the circumstances, somehow about 20 years have whipped by in a blur, and now it's you and your partner alone, together again at last. The autumn leaves are falling and the snap of winter is in the air at this point of your sexual life cycle.

At the end of the day, you sit across the table from each other and wonder who the familiar stranger looking back at you is. A long, long time ago, you were crazy about each other. Can either of you recall those special moments from early in your relationship—when all you had to do was just look at each other to start the juices of sexuality flowing? You peered into each other's eyes and everything your lover did turned you on. Those days—and nights—are now in the very distant past. Vacations for the past two decades were all about family, with infrequent smatterings of short you-two-alone opportunities to rekindle your sexual fires. Dinners for two required the logistics of babysitters and constant glances at your phone, calling in or texting: Did everyone do their homework? Did the baby finish dinner? Any trouble getting the younger ones to bed? As your kids matured, you watched for different types of texts. Did your newly licensed teenager make it to a friend's house safely? Is your daughter getting into a car with her boyfriend who's been drinking? Are they having sex without protection? Are they smoking weed at your house?

So much happened during the past two decades. Your marriage changed; sex and youth are no longer on your side. Remember the day you actually took your daughter to buy her first bra? How about the dress for her first prom? Did it even dawn on you that your time to play sex kitten was leaving, as you passed on the baton to the next generation? No one prepared you for the realities of parenthood and the transition from the vibrant, sexual being you were as a newlywed to the practically asexual middle-aged person you would become, as your role as a parent redefined you as a person.

For some of you, navigating your career track or climbing the corporate ladder took as much out of you as child-rearing. Work became all-encompassing, spilling into nights and weekends. Between parenting and the quest for success, your sex life fell through the cracks and you haven't seen it since. So when the two of you are finally alone again, a lot of contradictory emotions start to churn inside your heart and your brain.

Sounds terribly depressing, but it's only part of the picture, and we need to understand the entire picture to make life the best possible one at any age, so please stay with me.

MORE TIME TOGETHER MAKES FOR A BETTER MARRIAGE

A 2008 study published in the journal *Psychological Science* found that rather than heading for divorce court, more empty-nest couples experienced a higher rate of marital satisfaction, because they had more time together.[1]

LOSING THE SPARK

"This is not what I imagined my life would be like when we promised to love each other 'until death do us part,'" was my patient Stephanie's complaint. "When we got married at 27, we were such a hot couple. Sex was a huge part of what brought us together. I knew things would change, but I honestly thought our sex life was something we could always count on. When I first got married, I thought one of the perks was sex all the time. My husband told me that with us living together in a place of our own, we would be having much more sex than when I lived with my two roommates. He was right for a while. Three children, four moves, and more than a few economic ups and downs later, our sexual interest in each other has dwindled down to zero. I think about sex as something that might be fun with someone else; I'm not attracted to Adam anymore. He and I argue a lot about money and where we are at this point in our lives. I feel like calling this relationship still a marriage is a total misnomer. It seems more like an arrangement to me. I also think we are getting too old to even consider looking for other partners. Every guy in my age group is going out with women 30 years younger. If I leave Adam I will be alone—guaranteed!"

Sadly, Stephanie has hit upon a real and very sobering subject that affects too many couples. Marriages without sex are no longer the marriages they were when the couple got married. There is no doubt we need to redefine "marriage" at various ages and stop expecting the newlywed model to apply to couples married 15 or more years.

Until we universally change the definition of "marriage" at different stages in life, let's just try to understand the stages better. The marriage may still be working as a form of partnership, but, at some point, it might not be what you signed up for 20 or 30 years ago. Many patients tell me that life with their spouses is like living with a sister or brother or roommate. I cannot tell you how frequently I hear these analogies once the kids are out of the house and there are no friends or family to tell lies to or impress.

Many couples at this point in life have made a huge investment of time and emotion in their marriages. They had children, lived together for more than 20 years, and established their positions in life, and they identify themselves through the marriage and family they created with this partner. To the outside world, they often put on a show that things are always good and they are happy, yet behind closed doors the picture may not always be so rosy. Some couples are in cold-war mode, in which they barely speak. Some spouses argue constantly and can hardly stand each other's company. And of course they almost never have sex. These couples, whether they talk about it or not, have silently agreed to stay together for a multitude of reasons.

Money is the most common factor. Often the individuals in the couple can't afford to live separately. Maybe they're saddled with a second mortgage on the house or own a home that neither wants to give up. The most common reasons I hear for a couple's staying together at this point in life are children, grandchildren, and other family members. They worry that relatives will be shocked, hurt, or angry. Both partners are afraid of losing connection with the children, who often take sides when a breakup occurs. Sometimes, they're simply too embarrassed to admit to their community of friends that there is nothing left to keep them together. Despite the fact that 40 percent of marriages end in divorce, even the word alone—"divorce"—still carries the stigma of failure. Most couples want to save face. People are raised to care more about what someone else thinks about them than about how they feel themselves. There are implied and open pressures from culture, upbringing, social communities, and religious institutions for couples to stay together and celebrate 60 years of happy marriage. Finally, looming larger than life is the fear of being alone. Statistics in this area are scant, but the facts are only now emerging as more empty nesters are coming out and telling the truth about their marriages.

We all must take a hard look at our marriages long before the kids move out, if we want to avoid becoming a depressing statistic or if we are committed to celebrate honestly a long-lasting and fulfilling marriage. Often, by the time passion, respect, interests, and friendship have run out in a relationship, it may be too late to revive them. In those cases, the couple is better off admitting it and moving on. But unless you decide it's too late to salvage your relationship and courageously cut your losses, there may be time left for the two of you to rebuild a passionate, loving, and truly intimate bond. You must take advantage of this last chance to make it work before the two of you are left alone with one another, trying to avoid seeing each other in an empty house, wondering what went wrong. Start immediately by shifting the focus back to the two of you while the kids are still home, while you share that common bond, and while there's plenty of time ahead to redefine and rekindle the love affair. You *can* become intimate once again, even if your definition of "romance" has changed since your sex-filled honeymoon days.

Take the case of Priscilla and Joe, who were married for 19 years when their youngest son went off to college. Joe, 50, was an accountant working long and unpredictable hours, especially around tax time, when his clients needed him most. Priscilla, 49, was used to spending time without her husband. Having been a homemaker throughout the marriage, she was busy and satisfied with the kids, never noticing or minding that Joe spent most of his time at work. According to Priscilla, their marriage was good.

"Our sex life was healthy, full of fun and passion when we first got married, but over the course of about five years, it dwindled. There was less frequency and less passion—only about once a week—but I would still call it good sex," she told me when I first started seeing her as a patient. "Joe became more interested in work and the kids, and less and less sexual, and over the years, with the kids around and no time for each other, months suddenly started to go by without us even thinking of or having sex. Honestly, I didn't mind it, because eventually, I didn't care about sex either. I don't know if it was a reaction to Joe not touching me or to menopause, which started around the time the kids went to high school. None of my friends seemed to be having sex problems with their husbands, or at least they weren't talking about it, so I figured everything was normal.

"But once the kids were out of the house, I started to feel old. Suddenly, I was invisible. I remembered with sadness that when I was young, I'd felt highly sexual and always had the attention of men who thought I was hot. Lots of guys even tried to pick me up even after I was married. I never cared, because I loved my husband and wasn't interested, but I certainly enjoyed the attention. Now, I've put on weight and I am a size 16 when I used to be size 4 ten years ago. I feel unattractive, my life is boring, and Joe isn't doing anything to bring back the spark, so I feel taken for granted and horrible about myself. I just don't know what to do anymore. I went on diets and took pills that didn't work to help me lose weight; I hate exercising, and I'm feeling so depressed I don't really know what to do. I'm ready to go to the psychiatrist and get on antidepressants for the second time. The first time I took them, it was after my last baby was born and I was diagnosed with postpartum depression. But the truth is, I think I am depressed because I am just plain unhappy now and see no change for the better ahead. Maybe taking antidepressants will just dull my pain. It's either that or add a few more drinks to my ever-growing number of drinks at cocktail hour, as I've been doing over the past few years. I'm not alone there; all my friends in my age group are also drinking a lot more these days."

The awful truth is that many women at Priscilla's stage in life become depressed about both the loss of youth and the lack of sex in their marriages. Those who fake it and lie about how wonderful everything is between the sheets only serve to further depress those who, like Priscilla, are telling the truth and in search of a solution.

One day Priscilla came to see me in a panic. "I'm sure that Joe is having an affair with his secretary" she said, sobbing. When I asked her how she knew that, Priscilla told me, "He never notices me and comes home from work later than ever." I reminded her that she wasn't telling me anything new about Joe. He always came home late, and he didn't pay much attention to her even before the kids had left the house. This was the normal pattern of their relationship.

Priscilla thought it through and decided that I might be right, but the sudden possibility that Joe might have been cheating gave her the motivation to wake up and change her life. She not only wanted a real relationship with her husband, she wanted to have a passionate sexual love affair with him.

So Priscilla changed her approach. She started spending more time with Joe. She began to meet him for lunch, joined a local gym, and started working out regularly. Over a period of three months, without any drugs, she dropped 20 pounds. And most important, she started talking to her husband. At first, Joe was taken aback by the change in Priscilla. He had no idea how to relate to her. Suddenly, his wife was a different person. She dressed better and came up with lots of fun and sexy things for them to do together. Quickly, Joe responded in kind. It didn't take long for him to start bringing her flowers every week, something he hadn't done since they were newlyweds. She wrote him little notes and left them on his computer. In response, he started texting her love messages. When Priscilla suggested they go away for a weekend, Joe agreed, and while away at a resort, Priscilla and Joe rekindled their passion. There was more hot sex between them in that one weekend than there had been in 10 years. The passion, and with it the intimacy, was back. Priscilla and Joe conquered their empty-nest syndrome and came out on the other side with a worthwhile intimate and loving relationship—and sex to boot.

"Finally, we're happy, the two of us together. And the sex? Forget about once a week. Now it's more like three, and we're aiming for five!" Priscilla said.

FALLOUT FROM THE EMPTY NEST

Empty-nest syndrome is a real problem; more divorces occur as the last child leaves for college than ever before in the recorded history of marriages.

According to the American Academy of Matrimonial Lawyers (AAML), the divorce rate for baby boomers is rising. The AAML, with a membership of 1,600 attorneys, conducted a poll of its members recently.[2] The respondents reported an increase in the number of divorce cases in couples over 50 years of age. And while more men start divorce proceedings, 22 percent were started by wives.

A 2012 white paper from the National Center for Family and Marriage Research at Bowling Green State University in Ohio reported that while national divorce numbers have decreased in recent years, the divorce rate doubled between 1990 and 2010 for adults 50 and older. The change in numbers is dramatic: In 1990, fewer than one in 10 people over 50 were divorced. By 2010, that soared to more than one in four, which amounted to over 600,000.[3]

Yet there are solutions and possible ways to stem the tide. Eli Karam, an assistant professor in the Family Therapy Program in the Kent School of Social Work at the University of Louisville suggests that if you are married, you should:

- Create a long-term marriage plan that includes where you want to live and how you want to live your life as a couple. Most important, how do you see your marriage after the children leave? Don't wait until the last kid is out the door. Instead, start the dialogue when that child is in the first year of high school.
- Plan "protected time" each week when you do something together and then talk about it.
- Include your spouse in your interests (pastimes, hobbies).[4]

OTHER SCENARIOS

Sadly, not all stories turn out the same as Priscilla's.

"I've been married for 35 years," Lorraine explained. "I was very young, just 18, when we got married. Seth was 33 and already successful in business. Back then he liked to refer to me as his child bride. I always tried to take care of myself for him and, for 10 years before the kids left, I started going to a local medi spa in our town to get massages, Botox and fillers, and other antiaging therapies. Over the years, I became friendly with a female doctor who worked there. When I needed hormones to help me get through the menopausal transition, the spa doctor wisely placed me on bioidentical hormones. I felt and looked great. At one of the visits, the doctor mentioned that she also balanced the hormones of men who wanted to be able to keep up with sexy, youthful wives like me. She said she would be happy to consult and work with my husband, about his weight problem and lack of libido I'd been complaining for years about. Because I felt so at ease with her, I also confided about the loss of connection between Seth and me over the course of the years. I figured it was a combination of his intense focus on work and my involvement with the children. I thought the doctor's suggestion was so smart, because she thought hormone loss and aging could be the root cause of the loss of intimacy between us. Seth agreed, and over the next three years, things started to change.

"The treatments worked. He was truly rejuvenated and started to lose weight, went to the gym regularly, and even started getting checkups more frequently than once a year. But nothing really improved between us. In fact, he seemed to be away from home more than ever and rarely had anything to say to me when we were together alone. Our sex life never improved. The day we dropped our last child off at college, Seth announced he was taking me to a five-star restaurant for dinner. I was thrilled. I thought we were going to celebrate and begin a new, romantic phase of our lives. Instead, I couldn't believe what he had to say.

"Over dessert, Seth informed me he was leaving me. He said he had fallen in love with another woman and had waited for all the kids to leave before telling me he was going too. To say I was stunned is an understatement. I was so confused and hurt. Turns out the other woman was one of my best friends. We had raised our children together and she, her husband, Seth, and I went out together and even went on family vacations. I was so ashamed, I couldn't tell anyone, and I no longer trusted any of my friends. I felt everyone knew about it but me, and I was embarrassed to even go out. I couldn't go to therapy; I was too upset to talk, so I started drinking to dull the pain. My kids weren't very helpful. They blamed Seth and stopped talking to him, which initially made me feel vindicated, but it ultimately broke up the family I had worked a lifetime to build. Now that the kids have their own families, things have improved a little. But I still feel betrayed and sad.

"For me, life stopped the day Seth left. I know the truth is that we didn't have a good marriage, but it wasn't that bad either, and him having an affair with the woman I thought was my best friend is just unbelievable. I blame him but I also keep rehashing all the times I could have changed the course of our marriage, when I could have righted our ship—but I never really tried, because I just naturally assumed he'd always be there. I took him for granted, and he eventually left. It's now almost five years later and we are still tangled up in divorce court. I have finally found a therapist I trust, since drinking didn't ease the pain and only served to age me 20 years. I moved out of the old house I loved and am trying to make new friends in a new town I moved to, but at my age it isn't easy. I'm often frustrated and discouraged. Meanwhile, Seth is living it up. He married the other woman, all the children seem to have totally adjusted to the new family arrangement, and the friends we had as a couple accepted her as my replacement without a problem. Her husband disappeared after they got divorced. He moved back to Holland, where he was from.

"One of my children told me he thought he was raised in a big lie. He said he wasn't surprised this happened, since he always thought my husband and I had nothing in common and were just going through the motions of a pretend marriage. His comment made me feel even worse. I still can't understand what happened, but my kid has a point. I knew in my gut for decades that things were not right in my marriage, but I just ignored the problems. Sadly, I think I probably could've done something then. The end came anyway, but if I had been honest earlier, maybe we could've had a chance or maybe I would have left him first."

What Seth and Lorraine experienced is a sad but common ending to many long marriages. While the details are unique to each couple, the basic problems are similar. Passion and sex, along with whatever else seems like a good idea at the time, bring people together. They marry, have children and, throughout the rapidly passing decades of too much work, raising kids, and living life, they lose their connection. Their interest in one another falters, and when the kids are gone they split up, because one of them decides he or she no longer wants to be in the lifeless marriage they have. One or both realize their life is passing them by, and they want one more chance at happiness, sex, love, and passion, and their longtime partner no longer fits the bill.

SEXUAL TRANSITIONS, MARRIAGE, AND LIFE OUTCOMES

Most marriages start with a lot of sex, and the young couple equates the physical closeness of sex to a real relationship. When you are young and your future lies ahead of you, it's easy to jump into marriage without thinking what its foundation is and whether it will withstand the test of time. This is the spring of our sexual lives, and marriage is the natural progression toward our sexual summer. Once married, we enter the next phase of life. As the initial flush of sexuality starts to fade within several months—or, if you are lucky, years, the passion and intensity diminish; children and everyday life take over, and our sexual summer keeps us vacillating between being highly sexual and becoming less interested in sex while children and adult life issues take priority. These decades of raising children, working hard to create a nest egg, and even spending time enjoying our family lives represent the bulk of our sexual summer. While this time seems to last forever, in reality it passes by at supersonic speed, and it either brings two people together as a couple and helps lay a solid foundation to the marriage, or it divides a couple, leaving both people uninterested in one another between the heavy work of raising a family and the loss of the spark of sexuality. The marriage, the couple, the family, the jobs, the house, the lifestyle may look good to the outside world, but in reality too many marriages are lost in this transition; couples pay a huge price by having no relationship left to hold them together in the end.

The paths of partners' lives often diverge, as the years pass and the autumn of sexuality rapidly approaches. There are few options as time moves on and steamrollers over us. If there is real commitment and if the love that was initially manifested by great sex has matured and brought the couple together so that they like and accept each other and have fun together, the marriage will last. If, however, sex and intimacy are gone, and raising children is the only thing that is keeping the couple together, the marriage becomes an arrangement that is doomed and may not withstand the pressures of the outside world. As people enter the winter of their sexuality—menopause, andropause, and loss of visibility in our culture—most are left sad and afraid of getting old alone. In those very frequent cases, the marriage becomes an arrangement that may work for one or both of the partners so that they can maintain a facade to the outside world. Others may not be able to sustain the facade, and they split up, either looking to find new partners or simply preferring to live alone.

Loss of visibility and hence sexual status in our culture are the harsh reality of aging, and couples who are prepared and don't define themselves by the rules made by the outside world will survive, while those who haven't become real, intimate friends and partners will suffer the dire consequences of the winter of their sexuality.

The difficult and common truth is that often one or both partners are not truly committed to the marriage. In Lorraine's disastrous scenario, while she was focusing on raising her family and working hard at keeping up the happy family don't, her husband was not invested in the relationship, and since he was not having sex or getting enough attention at home, he started looking for love and sexual gratification outside the marriage. Sadly, many men and women follow this pattern predictably and consistently. When Seth began feeling and looking better and taking better care of himself, he started sending availability signals to other women. To find another man or woman willing to have sex and to listen to our tales of woe is too easy in our society. Seth fell prey to the easiest temptation: the sympathetic and bored ear and body of the woman next door.

There are many who believe that innocent flirtation keeps marriages fresh, and both men and women feel excitement and validation that keep them even more connected to their partners and the marriages, reassured of their continued attractiveness to others so they don't need to stray. Sometimes that is true, but all too often it isn't. In Seth's case, the flirtation led to sex and then—rejuvenated by a new relationship, passionate sex, and what he perceived as interesting company—Seth left Lorraine behind, relegated to a past he didn't even want to remember. Most people who make the decision to move on want to forget what went on before; thus, they don't learn or get better at creating a more substantial relationship the next time.

But there are so many other issues that must be addressed at this crucial crossroads.

WAS IT REAL WHEN IT STARTED?

Was he ever committed to her? Were Seth, Lorraine, and so many others who go through this transition and get divorced ever committed to the initial relationship? The answer is most likely yes. Most people don't just get married on a whim. The issue is that when you are young and get married, you aren't the same person you become as you accumulate years and experience. To define and expect the same thing out of marriage and sex at 50 as you do at 20 is plainly unreasonable.

Life takes so many twists and turns, and people's goals change constantly along the long and winding road of their lives. When I speak to patients who divorce after decades of marriage, they invariably tell me they were sure they loved their partner when they got married. But as time went by and the relationship started to disintegrate, they started to wonder if they ever did. I think most people do. I think most people start with good intentions, and in the fog of hormones and sex they realistically cannot see what 20 years out will look like. No matter what your parents or friends say, you are in the midst of a sexual and emotional frenzy that only you and your partner understand and participate in. It's easy to look at relationships and people from the outside and see their flaws and even predict potential outcomes, but the fact is, no outsider will ever understand what goes on behind closed doors in a marriage, and speculation and blame are a total waste of time.

WHEN IS IT TIME TO PULL THE PLUG?

I believe Lorraine probably did know at some point that her relationship with Seth was ending. Endings don't happen overnight. Like many people caught in the trap of infidelity regardless of gender, perhaps she was among the many who chose to see what they want to see—ignoring the obvious in the hope that it's just a phase that will pass. But the truth is that sweeping things under the rug never works. No one can survive living a lie forever without being deeply affected. So maybe you know a lot sooner than you are willing to admit that you no longer communicate with your spouse, that your sex life is no longer a passionate connection, or that, worst of all, you no longer care. But that may represent only a phase, since marriage and life are all about phases. If you really are committed to the relationship, you bite the bullet, confront the facts, and talk. But to communicate and get back into a loving sexual relationship once you no longer have it takes a lot of work and willingness to open up and be vulnerable and honest on both sides, at the same time. Help from marriage counselors may come in handy, but at the end of the day it boils down to whether you two really want to be together and work things out honestly as a couple. The only way to find out is to talk about it before one of you has strayed. Once the intimate act of having sex has occurred between one partner and a new one, it complicates the marriage and moves it faster toward its end.

EMPTY NESTERS: BY THE NUMBERS

In a 2017 study of 500 married baby boomers:

- 26 percent said they felt like newlyweds when their kids were out of the house, and even more (34 percent) stated they felt closer to their spouses without the children around.
- 58 percent said they were emotionally ready to get the kids out of the house. Males were significantly more likely to be emotionally prepared than females (70 percent versus 55 percent, respectively).
- 40 percent anticipated that their adult children would move back in with them.
- 30 percent anticipated that their parents would move in with them.[5]

When sexual attraction fades, intimacy disappears, and communication doesn't exist; when two people stay together because of responsibility toward family, children, financial entanglements, a house, and material things—that's the time when many people stray. Often, sad and lonely men and women seek out other relationships to get attention, to get validated that they aren't old and undesirable, and to bring some excitement into what they perceive as boring, sexless lives. It may be of interest to note here that in many cultures around the world and even in the U.S., it may become acceptable to stray; couples stay married and act as though they are still a couple in public, but behind closed doors where the only sound you hear is the TV, they are roommates or bedmates only. It's often just way of saving face, and it is what Jane chose.

"I took my vows very seriously. I was in love with Paul, and marriage was the normal next step in our relationship," Jane told me. "We were married almost 10 years before we had children. Hot sex wasn't the biggest part of our marriage even when we were young. Neither one of us had a big sex drive. Still, sex was good and we made an emotional and verbal commitment to spend the rest of our lives together in front of our families and friends. We married at 25, and now it's almost 30 years later. We raised the children together. Paul is a good father, and he always went to the kids' games, usually made it home for dinner, and was interested in everything the kids did. I worked in an office and made friends and always felt my life was good.

"A few years ago, I began to suspect that Paul was cheating on me. He didn't even try to hide it. When he went on business trips, he would add on a few days or even a week. Somehow, all his business trips started on weekends. I couldn't quite understand what business is conducted on Saturday night or Sunday, and if I asked he gave me vague answers. He almost always worked late. For my part, I knew things were stale, and the idea of sex with him had become a total turn-off to me over time. So my solution to knowing he was having sex elsewhere was to ignore it. In fact, it was a relief that he didn't want to have sex with me and wasn't asking for it. It was an easy out, and I didn't feel it was my fault. I am now in my 50s, I'm menopausal, and the kids are all gone. I will never leave Paul and I hope he won't leave me either. But you never know. I see everyone around me getting divorced as they get older, and it makes me wonder. Paul is a good guy and I have no more interest in sex, so he can have sex all he wants elsewhere. As long as he doesn't fall for one of his flings, I'm okay."

The number of women who talk to me so casually about this type of marital arrangement is surprising. Why do so many women feel it's okay to accept a loveless, disconnected relationship? Why do so many women feel they need to be married in our day and age? Most people just stay together because they are afraid to be alone. Dating as we age looks awfully grim, and the prospect of sex with a new man, taking off your clothes and letting a stranger see your aging body, is frightening and embarrassing to most women. Not to mention as men get older, the numbers of younger women finding them attractive keeps increasing.

"I was married at 20," Ellie told me. "I don't know why I was in such a rush, but Howard and I were so sexually charged, we couldn't keep our hands off each other. We had sex all the time. All I cared about was being with Howard. Our parents figured it was better we got married because they were afraid I'd get pregnant and then embarrass them and ruin my life. So they pushed us to get married. Since sex was the only thing we cared about and marriage meant legal, free, unprotected sex all the time, we jumped on the idea. We're together going on 30 years now. The first decade was great. Everyone around us was jealous of our overwhelming sexual attraction. While our friends' sex lives were dwindling, we were still going strong and there was many a morning we didn't make it to work on time after a night of many multiples of lovemaking. But that was then, and now I'm in another life.

"Slowly but surely things changed. I guess I shouldn't be surprised that we're not that attracted to each other anymore. He put on a lot of weight after he stopped being an athlete. He doesn't like to go out—I love to dance—and although he is a great dad and a good provider, I don't feel any kind of pull toward him any more. I'm a young 48; he's an old 49. He's losing his hair and he says he's tired all the time. There's no sex in our house. Neither one of us initiates or talks about sex. It's all a thing of the past. I resent him because he let himself go so badly. I know I really loved him and still do. I know I should be grateful; we made a lovely home and raised two good boys who are now married, and we have grandchildren and spend a lot of time with our families. I wouldn't want to be on my own; I see what happens when a woman gets divorced in this town. The minute she's single, she's no longer welcome to other people's homes and no one invites her to parties. If you dare split up, your social life is over. When you're not part of a couple, you're unwanted. I just couldn't live like that. But I am also having a hard time accepting my marriage the way it is now. It's like I'm living with my brother."

What should you expect from a good relationship, once the spring of sex and hormones has passed? To avoid becoming like Lorraine, Jane, or Ellie, you need to stay awake and alert during your life and pay attention to your own needs, your relationship, and your partner. Don't wait until the spark has gone out to start figuring out what intimacy means to you. Be honest all along and communicate.

CHANGING THE DEFINITION OF MARRIAGE TO FIT THE STAGE, THE PHASE, AND YOUR AGE

Marriage is a series of phases, ups and downs, and lots of changes that both partners go through, not always at the same time. As the years unfold and life moves on, are you allowing yourself to get bulldozed and flattened by age? Or will you make the best of each phase of your life? Many people tell me they want companionship and that sex is no longer a highly important ingredient in the marriage as they age. This is a different statement than defining a successful marriage on frequency and quality of sex, or concluding that a marriage is dead just because there is no more sex. At about the same time children go out the door to college and lives of their own, sex hormones are packing their bags as well. Husbands and wives must and certainly can find common ground as they move into this new phase. Memories are not enough to keep relationships vibrant. We need to look at ways to rekindle true connection and real friendship and to redefine a good relationship in realistic and workable terms. Redefining marriage at different stages is the key to success. If we use the same definition we used at age 20 for age 50, we'll fall short and feel dissatisfied and bored, and we'll start looking around for a better deal outside the marriage. Sometimes that may be the right thing to do—if you and your spouse have just grown apart, have nothing in common beyond parenting, or have moved so far away from the people you were when it all started. Otherwise, try working from inside the institution of marriage you created and spent decades on, and nourish it rather than demolishing it.

SOLUTIONS

- To prevent the empty nest from ending your marriage, you should:
- Take an honest look at the marriage and your expectations long before the children are gone. You need to know what you want to do when you no longer are raising a family and are just the two of you again.
- Seek marriage counseling, reconnect with each other, and rekindle or find new shared goals. Learn to listen to your partner and hear what he or she is saying.
- Make time alone for each other away from the children, the rest of the family, and friends.
- Don't hide at work; don't hide in a book, in front of a TV or an iPad, or on the phone. Just don't hide; face your partner no matter how tired or unhappy you are.

- Learn to communicate without anger, blame, or defensiveness. Learn to see the situation from your partner's perspective.
- Learn to accept and love one another for who you are now, not who you might have been or would prefer the other person to be.
- Don't stick your head in the sand when you know problems exist. Face the truth— cheating or lying or any other deception has to be confronted head-on when it happens, and you must decide what to do then and there. Things don't get better on their own; time doesn't fix anything. It only makes the burden of lying heavier. You must do the work to reap the benefits.
- Don't act as though everything is perfect just to save face.
- Redefine your values and what the relationship means to you.
- Do not follow our cultural definition of marriage. It doesn't apply to you, and it changes as you age. Don't fall prey to unreachable goals. Be gentle and accepting of yourself and your spouse.
- Don't treat your spouse with disdain; you've spent too many years together to end up in a cold war. Unless you truly have nothing left in common, it behooves you to find the commonality and enjoy each other.

- Laugh together and stop criticizing.
- Don't be submissive. It only serves to create resentment. All honest men want their wives to lead their marriages to success.
- Spend time together pleasing the other. Watch how fast you start feeling happier yourself and how quickly your partner starts noticing you and treating you well.
- Focus on how you behave in the marriage honestly, without "ifs," "buts," or "maybes."

CHAPTER 9

ANDROPAUSE, MENOPAUSE, AND SEX AFTER 50

"Male menopause is a lot more fun than female menopause. With female menopause you gain weight and get hot flashes. Male menopause—you get to date young girls and drive motorcycles."

—Rita Rudner

"Middle age? You've got to be kidding me! Fifty is the new 35," Lydia said. She has wavy brown hair without a touch of gray and a soft, beautiful complexion, with gentle smile lines around her eyes and mouth that make her even more interesting and attractive than some of my younger patients with smoother, fuller faces. Fit, energetic, and someone who lights up my office from the moment she walks in, Lydia doesn't believe in the ageist stereotypes that would relegate her to what our culture still terms "middle age."

"I love men. They love me. I don't want that to change. Why should it?" She came to me to help eliminate the bothersome symptoms of menopause, to keep her libido from plummeting, her vagina from drying up and her weight in check, and to start taking bioidentical hormones (the human identical hormones, which are the only hormones I prescribe).

Lydia is among a growing number of women—and men—who refuse to accept what previous generations took for granted: that hitting 50 starts the final descent into becoming invisible, asexual, old, and a member of AARP. When people have a healthier understanding of their bodies, when they focus on disease prevention and life extension, they learn that the right attitude, perspective, and health practices make the label and with it the entire concept of "middle age" null and void. While it is true that, for both men and women, hormones play a most critical role throughout life—in everything from sexuality to general health and well-being—it's also important to understand that times are changing and we now have the scientific evidence and practical tools necessary to keep both men and women vibrant and sexual for many more decades than in previous generations. It may be the beginning of the winter of your sexual life cycle, but winter doesn't have to be bleak or dead. It can be bright, crisp, and sunlit, with warm, crackling fires waiting for you.

SKIP THE LABELS, PLEASE

Traditionally, "middle age" has been defined as the beginning of sexual and physical decline, the era when balding men buy bright red sports cars and trade in their first or second wives for much younger models. Those abandoned first wives—so society's tired narrative would have us believe—are menopausal and depressed, except for the ones who go crazier than their husbands, running away from home and becoming "cougars." Or, having had enough of being ignored, they decide it's time to really live and start chasing after men younger than their sons, not unlike men who chase after younger women.

You may not want to read this, but even today, in 2018, according to the U.S. Census Bureau, if you are between 35 and 54 years old, you fit into the "middle age" category. Meanwhile, the Merriam-Webster dictionary defines "middle age" as the years between 40 and 60. From where I sit, "middle age" is a totally useless term in our culture, and it serves to make people panic and become depressed, thinking that the most productive years of their lives are consigned to their rear-view mirror. Nothing could be further from the truth.

While the medical profession is debating how to approach prevention of disease and sexuality as we age, there are millions of us in our fourth, fifth, sixth, and seventh decades and older who are finding these later years even more enjoyable and fulfilling than our youth. I'm not kidding, and it's not wishful thinking or rationalization. Wisdom combined with experience, optimum health, and enjoying life to its fullest, without little kids or the worries and drama of youth—that's a time for great fulfillment, not only the option to move into a retirement community and play bridge all day.

ANDROPAUSE

The media would have us believe that all men are sex-obsessed well into their older years. Hollywood abounds with images and the actual stories of 70-year-old movie stars with 20-something girlfriends and wives and little kids helping them hold on to youth and forestall mortality for another few decades. Such stereotypes land painful blows to many a woman's self-esteem, as they reinforce the idea that only a chronologically young woman deserves sex and male attention. Ironically, while doing the research for this book, I found out that the highest-priced, most exclusive matchmakers in general cater to rich older men and young women. There certainly is an overabundance of both. And still there are men who tell me they find that stereotype disturbing too. Many of them love their partners, and find them beautiful and desirable at any age. Many happy couples in their 50s, 60s, and later on like each other as they are, don't have to fantasize of younger bodies, don't turn off the light and pull the sheets over their faces when it's time for sex. Older men and women who love what they see as it looks and feels are usually those who have the most rewarding and truly intimate sex regardless of chronologic age. And, interesting to note, things often work out just great with younger men seeking older women when it's not just for financial security.

If you don't believe me, go to any online dating site (eHarmony, OurTime, EliteSingels, Match, Zoosk, and so on) and see how many 30-something-year-old men are looking to meet older women. Maybe it has something to do with knowing that older women are wise and experienced. They are less confused or confusing and more nurturing, and who knows? Maybe sex with an older woman could even be better from many a young man's perspective. You don't have very far to search to find these men; sometimes the leading man or the president of a country who has plenty of gorgeous young women available choses to go home to a woman his mother's age.

Men, just like women, go through a major life transition at this age; for them, it's called andropause (male menopause). During andropause, their hormone balance changes and the main hormone that defines manhood and males in general, testosterone, drops. Scientists have known about male menopause since the 1940s, but it wasn't statistically significant until male life expectancy levels rose enough for researchers to understand its importance and the need to address it.[1] Maybe because most scientists historically were male, they preferred to believe men were immune from menopause. In a male-dominated society, no one wanted to admit that when it came to aging and hormones, men were just like women. In the past, female menopause was obvious because an aging woman stopped getting her period and couldn't have children anymore, but many men never understood what was happening to their own bodies or just ignored any symptoms that might have belonged in the aging basket. Today, things are changing. Men are finally speaking out about the changes in their bodies, their moods, and even their libidos. Blood tests demonstrating significant drops in testosterone levels, a rise in sexual performance problems, the inability to build muscles, and the overall increase in male self-awareness are making andropause a fact of life.[2] Andropause is finally coming out of the closet and with it, a sea change in relationships between men and women.

Testosterone is a hormone both men and women make, only in different quantities. Women make a lot less, and men a lot more. Men make testosterone in their testicles, while women make it in their ovaries, and both genders make it in their adrenal glands (little glands on top of the kidneys). The importance of knowing this is that as men get older, their testicles tend to shrink. Along with the shrinkage on the outside, they make less testosterone on the inside. Men also make estrogen in small quantities, and the balance of estrogen and testosterone is very important; when correct, it keeps men healthy. When the balance shifts as men age, it causes problems not just with the hormones but also symptoms start to pile up. Besides being unable to sustain as strong an erection for as long a time as when he was younger, a man may experience weakness, fatigue, mood changes, reduced muscle and bone mass, thinning hair, increased body fat, and growing breasts. There are also increased incidences of high blood pressure, heart disease, and other chronic diseases of aging. The loss of testosterone directly affects men's sexual function and causes diminishing libido, loss of morning erections, inability to sustain erections, loss of duration and strength of erections, problems with ejaculation, and even impotence. Want to know some reasons why your formerly energetic and sexually obsessed husband is grumpy and lethargic? Most likely he's afraid of or plain uncomfortable talking to you about his flagging sex drive, so he would rather keep his nose in his book or be plopped in front of the TV or just get mad at you. It's not your fault his testosterone levels are dropping. But when it comes to reasons, it is his low testosterone that makes him feel old, afraid his good times are behind him, so unhappy, and sexually absent. Psychologically, men in andropause complain of depression, anxiety, irritability, insomnia, loss of memory, and reduced mental function. And they are unlikely to talk about sex, because they no longer can perform the way they did in their 30s. As a result, many men think it's best to just avoid the topic—and intimacy—altogether, which of course only serves to make marriages fall apart faster.

Testosterone Deficiency

- Low testosterone is associated with:
- Decreased muscle mass
- Loss of ability to build muscle
- Depression
- Weight gain
- Mood changes
- Increased fear of getting old and dying
- Loss of libido
- Loss of morning erection
- Erectile dysfunction
- Greater difficulty building muscle or just plain working out

Balanced testosterone (at 30-year-old levels) translates into:

- Great sex drive
- Positive outlook on the future
- Good weight control
- Easy muscle-building ability
- Strong and long lasting erections
- Good quality of sleep
- Morning erections

From the medical perspective, low testosterone is also associated with increased risk of heart disease and even Alzheimer's. The concern about a connection between testosterone and prostate cancer has overshadowed the positive effects of testosterone.

As a result, many physicians hesitate to prescribe testosterone to men who might desperately need it, and men still fear testosterone supplementation even if it does improve the quality of their lives. The entire debate over testosterone's fueling prostate cancer started in 1941 with a report in a medical journal about a patient with advanced prostate cancer and high testosterone levels. Even though much research has been conducted since then and the finding wasn't reproduced, the possibility of a connection between testosterone and prostate cancer still scares older men away from the use of testosterone. [3] To help dispel the misinformation, I strongly recommend reading Abraham Morgentaler's book *Testosterone for Life: Recharge Your Vitality, Sex*

Drive, Muscle Mass, and Overall Health. Taking medically super-vised testosterone in cream, gel, pellets or injectable form as they enter andropause and their testosterone production diminishes will greatly help keep men feeling and acting younger, as well as potentially prevent other diseases of aging—not to mention help save many a flagging sexual relationship. [4]

As andropause sets in and testosterone levels drop, sex drive plummets in many men. Lifestyle changes, environmental stress-ors such as health and money issues, as well as stale relationships at home worsen the problem. Often, environmental factors are used by men as excuses to avoid considering the possibility of low testosterone.

"I've always considered myself a highly sexual guy. I know I sound vain, but I know I'm good-looking, and women have been into me since high school," boasted trim, salt-and-pepper-haired Jason. "When we were very young, it really bugged my wife, Marie, when women would naturally flock to me anywhere we went. We had a lot of fights about it, but I always promised her and it's the truth—sexually, Marie was the only woman for me, and I was never unfaithful. Since the first night we spent together when we were barely 20, our sex life has been really fantastic. I talk to my married buddies about their sex lives, so I know we're among the lucky few—sex and passion have always been a big part of our marriage, and I'm sure it's one of the reasons our marriage is so solid.

"But when I hit 60, something changed overnight. My erec-tions starting getting unpredictable. In mornings I was no longer greeted with my consistently reliable erection. I must admit it scared me, and I saw a urologist, who checked me out and told me it was a normal part of aging. Not exactly reassuring. Who wants to be told that?

"When it came to sex, another disastrous chapter started. We'd begin serious, deep kissing and starting to touch each other, the usual great foreplay we had been enjoying for so long, and I'd immediately get a good erection—but by the time we got to intercourse, I suddenly would lose the erection. I thought if maybe we skipped the foreplay and got right to intercourse, that might solve the problem, but that turned out to be even worse. I never even got an erection anymore. Marie missed the closeness that foreplay gave us, and the "wham bam, thank you, ma'am" style of sex was never really my thing anyway. I couldn't perform on demand anymore. At first we tried to ignore it. But after a few months of frustration and embarrassment, I started thinking that maybe it had something to do with the medication I took for my high blood pressure. My doctor said there was no way the medication would cause my problem. He said it was my age and prescribed Viagra and later daily Cialis. We tried both, but I really hated them. Between the red eyes and the need to take a medication every day even if I didn't have sex, I felt like there was something wrong with me. It took me a while to figure out if I ate a fatty meal before taking the Viagra, I never even got an erection at all. The doctor never warned me. The drugs took all the fun and spontaneity out of our sex life.

"I started to get angry, which only lowered my libido even further. It wasn't getting older that bothered me—I'm in pretty good shape otherwise—it's just that so much of who I am was always tied into my ability to get it up whenever and wherever the mood strikes us. I couldn't talk about it with my friends. Trust me, guys only talk about sex when they're having a lot of it and can brag about it. Not one of my friends ever talked about not being able to perform. And the doctor I saw was useless; he told me there was nothing else I could do but take the drugs—or consider injections into the penis!

"One day, I was on an plane and picked up one of those magazines from the back of the seat. There was an article that caught my eye. It showed the picture of an older guy with a six-pack and all smiles promoting a medical clinic that catered to problems just like mine. It was a godsend. I made an appointment the next week. The doctor did blood and other tests and told me I needed testosterone. He prescribed weekly shots I learned to give myself. Within a day after getting my first shot, I felt like my old self again. In fact, I was so horny, all I could think of was sex within two weeks. I can't tell you how happy that made me. Now, a year later, the problem with sex is just a bad memory. My erections are great, and I am ready anytime I want to be. Marie and I have great sex again, and I feel 35."

VIAGRA: MIRACLE DRUG?

When Viagra came to market in 1998, it was a game-changer for both men and women. It was the first drug to help men get and maintain better erections, and while it was designed to help older men, it rapidly became the plaything of young men who wanted to see how long they could last with the addition of this medically approved, prescription sexual enhancer. It also brought sexual problems to the forefront and started a long overdue conversation.

"Erectile dysfunction" became the diagnostic label for this newly found "condition." Pfizer, the manufacturer of Viagra, had to make sure there was a diagnosable condition—so insurance companies would pay for its use. However, not all insurance companies fell for the ruse. Erectile dysfunction is really not a disease, and it turned out men will buy the drug, regardless of its exorbitant price.

Another issue with Viagra is that it's contraindicated for the very men who need it most. In older men with diabetes, atherosclerosis, hypertension, and cardiac disease, the inability to have and maintain erections is a symptom of their underlying atherosclerosis. The plaque causing atherosclerosis in the arteries of the heart is the same plaque that deposits in the arteries to the penis, since all arteries in the body are connected to one another. The blood flow is diminished due to the plaque in the arteries, thus leading to the loss of ability to get erections. The men with atherosclerosis are already at higher risk for heart attacks and strokes—and taking Viagra may even further increase that risk. In my view, Viagra and its cousins, Cialis and Levitra, also fail in their ability to help men who are depressed and have no libido to begin with. It's one of those typical pharmaceutical solutions to treating a symptom, not addressing the root cause, and creating more negative side effects in the process.

As I mentioned above, there's one great thing that Viagra has done for men and those who treat them as they age—once it came to market, suddenly everyone was talking about the formerly taboo subject of sex and the aging man! Celebrities and even the likes of politician Bob Dole promoted Viagra in nationally aired TV ads and admitted to having problems with erections. This brought the entire issue of flagging male libido out of the closet and helped millions of aging men realize that they're not alone with this problem. So thank you, Viagra!

FADED ATTRACTION

A day doesn't go by without a patient telling me that he or she no longer finds their partner sexually desirable. This situation is not just hormonally driven; it also is a reality of long-term relationships that few want to talk about. It's a lot more common than you think. After decades of marriage, a large majority of couples find themselves living like brothers and sisters or as roommates in pretty much asexual relationships. The truth is that most humans do get bored having sex with the same person for decades. Not many want to talk about it, and if you add chronic illnesses that come along with aging, plus the humdrum of everyday existence with another person, intimacy changes from sex to just doing your own thing under the same roof as your spouse. Sometimes things work out simply because the two people become best friends and share life experiences; they travel, work, and raise kids together, have grandchildren, experience losses and successes, and of course have all the holidays and family and friends and gossip. Not everyone strays; many lose interest in sex altogether, and that is just fine. My patient Harry is a typical example.

"June and I got married right out of college," Harry, 57, told me. "Over the years, like other couples, we've experienced lots of ups and downs. Now we're sandwiched, with our daughter back from college and living at home with us, taking care of June's father and my mother. They still live on their own nearby, but basically one of us is over there doing something for them every day. It's a lot to handle, plus both of us still work. Personally, I'm stressed all the time. We used to look forward to a retirement where it was just the two of us, but now that's been put off indefinitely.

"I still love June deeply, but the weight on her shoulders has taken a huge toll. She's just as beautiful to me inside, and when we get a moment to come up for air and go to a movie or out to dinner, we really enjoy each other's company. But when I look at her, I see an old, tired woman, even though she's only 55. I hate myself for being so superficial, but it's true. I know that I'm no catch either, but I was always the one to initiate sex in our relationship, and lately I'm not interested because I just don't feel as attracted to her as I used to. When we occasionally do have sex, it's okay, but frankly, I'd rather masturbate if I feel the urge than have sex with her. How can I talk about it with her? I mean, I'd sound like the biggest asshole on the planet. It's not like I'm going to run out and find a 25-year-old mistress—I don't want that either. I just wonder if this is simply the end of the road for us as a sexual couple. Maybe that's just fine. Too bad no one talks about it or tells us not to worry about it, that we are normal."

Sexual attraction is a mysterious thing. Harry and June are more typical than most of us admit. Is there hope for them? As long as we are alive, there always is hope. However, if we genuinely feel the sexual part of our marriage is over, maybe it's time to admit the truth and redefine companionship and friendship as the relationship's new normal. At the very least, those in long-term relationships need not compare their sex lives to what they see in the media, to their own sex lives at 35—or to those who profess to still have hot sex at 70 with their spouse of 50 years. Everyone is different. Maybe if we become honest with one another and let each one of us define what's right for us in a relationship, we may be able to create a different but still solid marriage that may happily and satisfactorily last for the next 40 years.

Or maybe it *is* time to admit you want something different. Some people truly and honestly can't live without sex in their lives, no matter what their chronological age, and some relationships just run their course and do end. It doesn't really matter how much you loved your partner when you got together or how old you are when you decide to split up. Most people are looking for validation and security, and sex very often defines how we feel about ourselves, and is a need that might have to be satisfied even in our later years. If both parties involved are honest, there is always room for a compromise out there. At the end of the day, you have to decide what matters most to you—it's your life, after all. You can chose honesty, communication, and a real, intimate relationship; you can choose to let go of sex as a primary determinant of intimacy and work on creating intimacy from your joint history, life experience, and friendship; or you can just save face and pretend. It's all up to you.

MALE MENOPAUSE BY THE NUMBERS

- In 1950, less than 5 percent of the world's population was older than 65 years of age.[5]
- In contrast, by 2025, more than 15 percent of the world's population will be older than 65.[6]
- The number of men in the United States who are 65 years of age is projected to increase from 14,452,000 in 2000 to 31,343,000 in 2030.
- Approximately 30 percent of men ages 60 to 70 and 70 percent of men ages 70 to 80 have low bioavailable or free testosterone levels.[7]

I have a patient named Eric, in his early 60s, whose solution to his flagging interest in his wife was to get divorced and set out on a quest for sexual variety.

"I left Carol 10 years ago; though it was painful at the time, I knew it was the right thing to do. The truth was, our sexual relationship had been dead for decades and I just didn't want to live like a monk for the rest of my life. Since then I've never gone lacking for female company. When I see an attractive woman, sex immediately comes to mind. It's not very different than when I was young. I date several women at a time, and I believe this keeps me interested in sex and interesting to women. From my own and other men's experiences, I know what happens when you have sex with the same person for a long time. It invariably gets boring, and you lose interest and then lose your erections. I don't want to sacrifice my sex drive, because I think if I do, I *will* get old, and it's not something I want to give in to. There are always so many women, even more now that I'm older; I feel like a kid in a candy store. I like tasting every candy. And if I need a little help from the pharmaceutical industry, I'm fine with that, and no one has ever complained about it to me."

My patients also include men who never married but who are still searching for the right woman. Their perspective on sex over 50 may seem unusual but is worth noting. Whenever Rob, 63, comes into my office, he brings me up to date on his latest conquests. He loves to go on cruises and take trips, because he likes sex without having to get involved in long-term relationships.

"My most recent trip was a Pacific ocean cruise," he told me. "There are always more solo women than men on the ships, so I get to choose who I want to pursue. I usually pick a pretty woman, and most of the time it turns out they are divorced or widows. I ask them to go out for coffee, and then we start spending time together. We always have a good time, with trips ashore and sightseeing and meals together. It's easy and romantic. Do we really get to know each other? I can't really give you a solid answer on that one. It's like a short, fun relationship on fast-forward. It's a great fantasy. We are both adults, and we both understand it's just about sex. Once we get home, there are usually geography issues, not to mention the fact that more than once I hooked up with women who turned out to be married or engaged or otherwise taken. I guess what goes on at sea, stays at sea. Even if once in a while I meet a woman whose company I truly enjoy and sex is really good, inevitably the romance ends when the ship docks. Still, the trips are great and totally satisfying to me. I get to see new places and meet new women. It makes me feel forever young. I love this life and wish I had started living it 20 years earlier. I doubt any of the women I meet expect anything more than just a fling, given the circumstances. It's fun for both sides and it doesn't do any harm."

There is nothing to say about Rob without passing judgment. He is happy; he certainly doesn't seem to be doing any damage to himself. Rob's life is working just fine for Rob. And hopefully the women he courts on his trips are adults and should be able to figure out what he's all about and not develop fantasies of permanence.

Then there is the classic story of the aging husband who leaves his wife for a much younger woman. We may call it a midlife crisis, but it happens at all ages and for many reasons.

William is a successful 65-year-old who has been married three times to younger women. He is a mogul at work and collects Porsches and modern art. He also collects young women. His latest is a 23-year-old girl he met in a bar during one of his business trips. He brought her home and within two months married her. When I asked William what he has in common with her, he smiled and said: "Sex. She looks at me as a father with benefits, and she is so grateful I am giving her this magical life. All she has to do is spend my money to dress well and sexy and be on call for all my sexual needs when I want it. I know she's happy, and I don't care if she's in love with me or not." The women seem happy and William is certainly happy too—another perfect example of living in the moment without long-term responsibility or accountability.

WHERE DOES THAT LEAVE THE MIDDLE-AGED WOMAN?

Many of my female patients come in with this story. They were married for decades to men who treated them poorly all along, yet they never gave up hope or considered leaving the marriage. When they were young, the men went out with their buddies one too many nights, there were one too many business trips, they didn't really help with the kids, and they were stingy with their financial and/or emotional support, always focused on themselves first, and when the wife asked for help, they'd growl, "I'm the breadwinner. I don't need to do anything else." All too often these are the kinds of guys who leave a potentially salvageable marriage in the quest for eternal youth, leaving the abused and emotionally beaten-down wives blaming themselves. These women come into my office and say things like, "I'm not as attractive as I used to be. I can't compare with a bikini-clad 20-something-year-old. It's totally my fault he left, because I've been a nag for decades. Who wants to be with an old woman? I don't really blame him."

This is not a pretty picture, but it is what I see and hear too often. Subservient women who devote a lifetime to self-absorbed and uncaring men and yet expect the marriages to work out and the men to stay with them to the end.... What is wrong with the women? Once you figure out a man is selfish and not a partner, why stay with him?

I hear the reasons: "No one gets divorced in my family" (or, "My parents got divorced, so I swore I'd never do that to my kids"), "We have kids together; we made a beautiful family together; we've been together too long for me to move on; I still hope he'll come around if I just do one more thing better...." These women make it very clear they need help building self-confidence to get out of these situations long before they are discarded for newer models.

Let women like Leslie be the example of the new middle-aged woman we should emulate.

Leslie is 64. At 59, she left a 30-year relationship because it was stale, she was more successful than her partner, he couldn't keep up with her, there was no sex, it depressed her to be around her couch-potato man, and she knew she didn't want her life to just pass by while she impotently watched the relationship die out. She moved out and spent a year developing new skills. Leslie knew she wanted to be alive. She knew she wasn't done with men, nor was she ready to just go out with her friends who had closed the book on romance and sex. She hadn't dated since college, so she prepared herself to start dating again. She got a coach, worked on her self-confidence, read a few self- help books and got into great physical and mental shape. After a while, she joined online dating sites, put together her profiles, posted some great pictures, and was off to the races. Her life changed dramatically. She says she's having the best time of her life. She meets interesting, successful, healthy, and exciting men who provide her life with more texture and fun than she had in college. She says it's more fun to date in your 60s, because you are wiser and more experienced and you enjoy sex even more than in your 20s. But don't think Leslie is the female version of Rob. She is very clear that she is looking for love, for a true partner to get old with, a man to have passionate sex with who is her intellectual equal and friend. Leslie is the perfect role model of successful dating with a clear end goal.

In fact, when people are dating in their 50s, 60s, and older, sex becomes very important again and intimacy is easier to attain if both the man and woman have the same goal of finding ever-lasting real love.

Regardless of how you get there, whether you follow the Leslie model or stay in a marriage for life, the outcome should be one of mutual satisfaction and success.

Take the couple I will call the Smiths. She is about 70, and he is in his mid-60s. They are both gorgeous people. They have been together for 45 years. They have three kids and 15 grand-kids. They live in the same house they raised their children in and do everything together. They care about each other, and she tells me in front of him that when she sees him pulling into the driveway from a window in their home, her heart still goes pit-ter-patter. When I asked them why their marriage has survived and even thrived, they gave me a few answers we all need to pay attention to. They even teach young couples at their church about how to have solid and long-lasting relationships. And they are great at it. Their advice is simple and works:

1. They like each other.
2. They laugh together.
3. They have common interests—in their case, they sing and dance together, are elders in their church, and travel on missions together.
4. They genuinely care to spend time together, and they are not afraid of getting old.
5. They say they like being old together. It's more fun because they have memories and a lifetime they've shared and so much more to look forward to together.
6. They don't have unreasonable expectations of each other. They accept each other's flaws with smiles on their faces. They like each other's bodies as they are now—full of wrinkles and sagging skin, love handles, you name it.
7. They don't hold grudges, and they talk everything through.
8. They have a lot of sex. By that I mean once a week since they got a little older, but with the help of hormones, some pharmaceuticals, and each other's support and love, and always remembering to be touchy and feely, they have managed to keep sex alive and well in their household.
9. They behave like teenagers when I see them together. They giggle and flirt with each other.

10. They focus on each other and their relationship above everyone and everything else in their lives. They are generous of spirit and financially, and they love their kids and grandkids, but above all else, they truly love each other.

I wish I could reassure you that this is the way most couples I see in my practice grow over the years. But when patients come into my office, I can also tell when they are altering the truth to suit what they perceive my expectations to be. I've heard female patients place 100 percent blame on their husbands for the fact that the men left them for greener pastures, when that is never the entire truth. It may not just be aging and lack of sex that drove the husbands away. Maybe when the women started focusing on having kids and growing their families, they put their husbands on the back burner and left them there. Maybe they stopped being interested in having sex and did everything they could to keep them away. Maybe they nagged the men and subtly put them down to disguise their own disappointment with their husbands as partners, instead of working to get them on the same page when they were young. Life is a continuum, and our behaviors from our 20s have consequences forever.

Or maybe it was the men who treated the wives poorly and put them down for years, but the women never had the courage to tell them how they felt. The husbands came to think of their wives as doormats and eventually got bored and moved on. Self-blame never works, but we can't move on unless we face the truth and take responsibility for marriages that don't work. Thus, the past becomes our teacher, not our jailor. The best way to move forward is to take to heart the lessons of our past experiences and attempt not to repeat the same mistakes. As long as we are alive, we have another chance.

When I was in my mid-40s and recently divorced, one of my friends wanted to set me up with a guy who was in his 50s. I was never one to date a lot, so I asked her a few questions about him before considering going out with him. One of my questions was, "What age group does he usually date?" Her answer was, "He likes really young women, but you look so great and are a successful professional, so he should be okay with your age." I told my friend to forget about the guy immediately. If an older man prefers young women, he will never be interested in a woman his own age. And why would I ever want to be with someone who wouldn't want to be with me? You should only be with someone who wants to be with you!

Our culture seems to accept and encourage powerful, confident men to be with much younger women. For decades, if an older woman went out with a younger man, she was the subject of ridicule. But all that holier-than-thou attitude went out the window when 70-year-old celebrities began parading around with 20- and 30-year-olds on their arms.

I believe things are changing. At the 2014 Golden Globes, Tina Fey and Amy Poehler joked about the blockbuster outerspace drama *Gravity*, starring 52-year-old George Clooney and 49-year-old Sandra Bullock. "*Gravity* is the story of how George Clooney would rather float away into space and die than spend one more minute with a woman his own age," Fey said. The audience went wild with laughter. Comedy is a sneaky way of telling the truth to those who might not be able to tolerate it any other way.

But is attraction to a younger body the whole story? I don't think it is.

When I was in my 30s, I worked at a hospital with a physician who notoriously married a new younger woman every decade. One day, I asked him the reason why. He gave me an interesting answer that still holds true almost 30 years later. He told me, "Younger women expect very little from older men. They are so happy to be with a man who is financially stable, appreciates their bodies, and isn't all that interested in their minds. It makes for an easy relationship.

"Older women, wives, women you go through long periods of your life with are difficult. They want to be partners, they want to know what you are thinking, and they have expectations from you. Sex loses its attraction when the rest of the time you are with a nag and a torturer. Men don't want to be bothered."

This physician may have been claiming he speaks "the brutal truth all women need to hear," but listen between the lines to what he's really saying about himself. In the worldview of this doctor and men like him, intimacy equals high expectations and work. One of the things I hear repeatedly from both men and women who admit to being unfaithful is that someone they have a brief affair with doesn't have time to find out enough about them and that is a good thing. A new lover won't nag them, judge them, or expect very much from them. Ideally, we all seek the fantasy of unconditional adoration from our partners. Isn't that why prostitution still exists? Prostitutes are women who just have sex and never ask for anything except money. Unfortunately, with that approach the only way a person can get truly unconditional love is from a dog. And that's a totally different story.

My doctor colleague takes the easy way out by never addressing things he might have to improve in himself in order to have a long-lasting relationship, by choosing young, easily infatuated women who always look up to him as perfect—or at least tell him so. Of course, we all deserve to be loved for who we are and not mercilessly criticized. But a man who is a serial husband, marrying increasingly younger women as he ages, is cheating himself out of the opportunity to grow up and deal with his fear of simply being human and being seen for who he really is. He's unwilling or just unable to have an intimate relationship of the heart and mind.

MENOPAUSE

We know that women lose their sex hormones as they age, just like men. By the time the kids reach puberty, their mothers are starting to experience hot flashes, night sweats, insomnia, irregular periods, and weight gain. Slowly but surely, women enter menopause, that time of life when they are no longer fertile, and estrogen, progesterone, and testosterone production diminish significantly, eventually disappearing altogether. While research on hormones and their roles in women's lives has been going on since the late 1800s, little was written about it and even less was talked about until only 20 years ago. Unbelievably, even today medical schools don't provide any significant or up-to-date training on the subject of menopause and the use of hormones in wellness and disease prevention.

Physicians who should be resources in the area of hormone therapies and treatments for menopausal women are polarized between the pro- and anti-hormone schools of thought, leaving women without the much-needed support hormones provide to protect them during this new phase in their lives. Sadly, postgraduate medical training doesn't provide balanced or useful information, and compassionate, reassuring care is scarce at a time when women need it most.

Menopause is a significant passage in a woman's life. It signifies the end of the periods she's had since her teens and the end of her fertility—both characteristics that help to define her. For most women, menopause is a confusing time, leading to a permanent loss of identity.

Historically and anthropologically, not too long ago women did not live long past their childbearing years—even if they survived childbirth, they rarely lived long enough to enter menopause. As a result, not much was known or spoken about it. As women started to live longer and most started reaching menopause, they hit another huge stumbling block to education and empowerment: cultural taboos and control by men and society over women's bodies and minds. With the rapid advances in medicine and science and the industrialization of our society, as life expectancy grows still longer, women's roles after menopause are changing dramatically and must be addressed and studied seriously and without prejudice. Women's wisdom and experience, when coupled with well-balanced hormones and healthy living, can quickly turn an erstwhile disposable old woman into a smart, sexually turned on, and worthwhile contributor to society.

MENOPAUSE BY AGE

All women who live long enough will enter menopause. **Natural menopause** usually occurs between 45 and 55 years of age. The average age for menopause is 51.

The average age of the onset of menopausal transition is 47.5 years, and the transition to the next phase lasts four to five years.

Late menopause (after the age of 55) occurs in 5 percent of women.

Early menopause (between ages 40 and 45) occurs in 5 percent of women.

Premature menopause, or "premature ovarian failure" (before the age of 40), is experienced by approximately 1 to 2 percent of women. It is caused by environmental, genetic, surgical, or chemical factors (IVF, chemotherapy, and so forth).[8]

The journey through menopause is different for every woman. Some tell me that the experience isn't as difficult as they expected. Others say that it's a horror show. Many say it happens suddenly, while others say it's a gradual process that takes years to unfold. Some women tell the truth about their experiences, while many don't. While menopause doesn't carry with it the same stigma it once did, too many women are still afraid to talk openly about it because they are afraid of being labeled as old. It's a shame, because the more we talk and understand this natural biological transition, the more comfortable women can feel about the aging process and the less they'll feel limited by it. There are still many women who lie about their age out of fear of being perceived as old in our youth-obsessed culture.

Ageism is the bane of our society, and "old" is still a socially derogative term affecting both men and women.

My three decades of working in the wellness field, focusing on optimum lifestyles for longevity and disease prevention, have shown me again and again that every individual is different, physically, emotionally, and of course sexually. Balancing hormones may help prevent disease and keep us functioning optimally as we age, but the way we respond sexually is not driven by hormones alone. As I mentioned at the beginning of this book, other factors come into play, and to ignore their importance is to do us a disservice and miss the point. While every one of us is different and all women experience menopause and every other phase of life differently, there are common threads we must find to bring us together and help us feel less alone and more empowered as we navigate the choppy waters of life.

MENOPAUSE AND THE BODY

Carly, 52, related her experience to me. "No woman in my family ever told me what to expect, but I do remember overhearing my mother and my aunt whispering about being 'dried up' at some point while I was young and totally naive," she said. "I didn't have a clue what they were talking about. As an adult, I never thought about menopause. In fact, I never heard anyone talk about it. Suddenly, when I started experiencing hot flashes and severe night sweats, I thought I was dying of some horrible disease. I went to my doctor, who dismissed me with a pat on the back and told me, 'You're just menopausal, honey. It's a normal part of aging.' His reaction didn't make me feel better. In fact, I left crying that I was now old and useless. I went home and Googled "menopause," and it opened a whole new world of information and chatrooms for me. Sharing the information and reading other women's stories were such a relief to me, because it made me feel I was normal and I wasn't alone or just plain roadkill.

"Initially, I figured I could just ride out the symptoms, but their strength and frequency kept increasing. The hot flashes felt like my head was in an oven all day, night sweats kept me changing sheets and pajamas all night. For the first time in my life, a spare tire started to develop around my middle. Then one day I woke up and realized I hadn't thought of sex for weeks and couldn't care less if I ever had it again. That's what you call 'loss of libido.' It's also when I remembered the 'dry' reference and made the connection with my mother's menopause. But I am an intelligent and successful woman and I like sex, so I decided that if I didn't have to put up with these symptoms, I wasn't going to. I came to see you and started taking bioidentical/human identical hormones, and all my symptoms disappeared, practically overnight. To specifically help with my libido, you gave me testosterone and a vaginal cream with hormones in it. I've told you before but I want everyone to know. You gave me my life back. My sex drive came back, and my husband and I found ourselves enjoying sex again like we did 20 years ago. No kids around and no concern of getting pregnant. Freedom indeed. Our marriage has never been sexier or more fun."

And Carly is not alone. There are many patients I see who find menopause a source of renewed freedom. Beth, 51, explained it very well.

"No more birth control! I've been sexually active since I was 17, and I've always loved sex," she said. "However, over the years there has always been a damper on my sexual freedom—whether it was fear of getting pregnant when I didn't plan on it, getting my period every time we went on a romantic vacation, or just having to organize my sex life around periods. The moment my periods ended, I felt free and happy. I never missed it for a second; no more bloating, PMS, or cramps. I never understood why so many women literally mourn the end of their period or go on hormone regimens that keep them having periods into their 60s. I don't need a period, and my sexuality is not tied into carrying a label, menopausal or not. This is the best time of my life. Sexually and emotionally I feel on top of the world. I am taking bioidentical/human identical hormones because I know they are keeping me lubricated and very sexual, and they are keeping my brain sharp and my body looking good. There's nothing more I can ask for!"

Shortly after the publication of my book *The New Hormone Solution*, I was giving a talk in New York City. As I talked about hormones, menopause, and sex, a woman in the audience raised her hand. She was in her 50s and said she wanted to thank me for giving back her life and her vagina. Another woman chimed in and said since she had been taking bioidentical/human identical hormones, her vagina felt like it was 20 again. The first woman interjected, "My vagina feels like it's 35." I was stumped and asked what was the difference. She said a 35-year-old vagina enjoys sex more than a 25-year-old one. It's all about experience. The entire room burst into laughter.

The experience was fun for the audience, and I loved seeing both men and women nod their heads in agreement. I felt a sense of fulfillment about the work that is my passion—I was helping women and men stay healthy and happy as they aged. What these people were saying was that sex gets sexier with age.

SEX AFTER 50: WHAT TO EXPECT

Lots of women still see their sex lives change, or even end, once they enter menopause and in the years that follow.

"When my marriage ended, I knew I wanted to remarry," Sonia, 58, told me. "For one thing, my ex remarried within a year. For another, I'm not a woman who's meant to live alone. To me, having a companion to go through life with seems like the way life should be. It's all about sharing your life with another person.

I tried online dating, setups, trips, courses, groups…you name it. So far I haven't met the right guy, but I am confident it will happen. More than a few guys made it perfectly clear that they would be glad to have sex with me but they weren't looking for 'commitment.' I know I am. Even at this age, though, I know the right guy will come along and sweep me off my feet. Ironic, isn't it? It's like being in my 20s all over again. There is something attractive and sexy about feeling this way! And it probably wouldn't be if I wasn't taking hormones and feeling good about myself."

Another patient of mine, Nicole, also 58, told me, "I'm happy with my life and my husband of 35 years, but I keep it interesting by always having a little innocent flirtation going on. Whether it's a guy at work or a friend from the distant past, someone I meet in the street or at a convention, I just notice them and they notice me, and the little glance or the little smile suffices to keep me feeling sexy and interesting. I don't have sex or become intimate with any of them, but it keeps me from feeling invisible. Getting just a little sexual attention from other men helps me get turned on to my husband as well, and I'm convinced that's why I still find him sexy and we still have hot sex, even after all these years."

Bravo, Nicole! More women should learn from her example. She keeps herself feeling attractive and sexual without hurting anyone. She keeps her home fires burning strong because she feels good about herself, and that is with the help of hormones and her great attitude.

While Nicole is active and sexy and Sonia is still searching for the man of her dreams, other women are fine with closing the door on the sexual parts of their lives.

"The love of my life died over 10 years ago," Elena, 65, told me. "We were married for 15 years, definitely the best time of my life. I know that I'll never find that kind of intellectual and physical connection again. So the end of my sex life doesn't bother me. What Nick and I had was special. He was my second husband, and we had passion and fun. I know he was my soul mate, and I am happy I had the time with him. I can easily live the rest of my life with the wonderful memories of the amazing connection we had. There are so many other ways I can be a contributor to the world; to me it doesn't have to include sex. I teach and belong to numerous groups that travel doing humanitarian work all over the world. I feel my life has purpose, and I don't need to change it for now."

Other scenarios unfold differently.

"After 28 years of marriage, I finally walked out on Ed," Laura, 59, related to me. "He was a serial cheater, and I stayed with him much too long. First I fooled myself into thinking I should stay for the kids. Once the kids were gone, I stayed just for the family and friends. But once I hit menopause, something shifted in me. It's like my body told my mind, "Enough with the lies." All of a sudden, I didn't care what other people thought anymore. I couldn't stand being with him. The divorce was rough financially for both of us. Ed still had his well-paying career, but I'd given up my banking job decades before to raise the kids. I had missed my opportunity to have a career, so I've only been able to find a part-time job for a nonprofit agency. I also ended up with a lump-sum division of our shared property. But I was at the point where I didn't care about money; I just wanted out.

"Within a year after the divorce, I met Dave through friends. He was retired, a few years older than me, and was estranged from his family. Like many men, he hated being alone and wanted to have a woman to make a home for him. I certainly was in a position where I could use economic support, and as we became friends, we came to an agreement. We would move in together, I would make a home for him, take care of him, and he would pay the mortgage on the house we both shared. It was always clear to both of us that sex was not a priority and if it happened, it would be a bonus. He agreed. It's not a bad arrangement, and we get on really well. It's not a passionate love match, but it works, and I am happier and more at peace than I was either living with my husband or alone. And when it comes to sex, we do it once in a while and it feels like a treat. I'm really happy with my life."

SEXUAL ACTIVITY AMONG OLDER WOMEN [5]

	Age 50–59	60–69	70–79	80+
Masturbated in previous year	54%	46%	36%	20%
Had intercourse in previous year (penis–vagina)	51%	42%	27%	8%
Had oral sex in previous year	34%	25%	9%	4%

Some married women also decide to retire their sexuality.

"I believe our marriage is solid," Linda said. "But after 40 years together and three grown children, financial worries, medical issues, my menopause, his menopause, neither of us wanted to take hormones. We decided to just age naturally, and now we don't care about sex at all. We talk, we laugh and spend a lot of time together, and we are happy. I hope he isn't lying about his side of the sex story. I would hate to find out he's got a young chick on the side, although as long as it's for sex and not love, it might not be a deal breaker for me at this point in my life. I do believe we have a good life and our lifetime of memories cannot be erased by any one-night stand he might have had. I live for today and enjoy his company—even without sex."

THE CHOICE IS YOURS

My mother used to say, "Aging is not for sissies." Others would say, "It's not for the faint of heart." When I was in my 20s and 30s and even 40s, those words seemed silly, and I didn't understand what the big deal was. Then suddenly, it was my turn to hit 50, then 60. Seemingly overnight, I had joined the ranks of the "middle-aged," even though I felt (and still feel) 35. But experience and listening to my patients have certainly prepared me for this time of life. In our youth-obsessed culture, we're sold on the idea that sexuality and excitement in life are only for the young. I can definitely say—as a doctor and a woman—that nothing could be further from the truth.

Sexuality does indeed change as we age. While during our teens and 20s it may represent the sum of our lives' focus, things change a bit as time goes on. With the passing years, sexuality comes to represent only part of the entire picture that makes up our lives. As the impact of hormones diminishes, life gets busy and relationships settle in, and the importance and desire to have sex pale in comparison to the importance they had in our youth. Sometimes a new version of sexuality replaces it, and sometimes sex leaves the scene altogether. But even that's not necessarily a negative. We have a choice: Obsess over what we've lost or rejoice in the greater gifts we've gained. Those who spend the time doing some honest soul-searching discover that while aging brings us closer to life's end, it also brings richness in wisdom and experience, and more appreciation of everything we have.

I've watched so many of my patients at this age come to relationship crossroads, only to do the necessary hard work and come out stronger than they could have ever imagined. Done right at this age, relationships can deepen and thrive. Sex becomes much more forgiving, more intimate, even more playful and relaxed than when we were young. On the other hand, if both parties can admit that a relationship is really over, it may be time to move on. The decades or years you have left ahead of you are more precious than ever, and both you and your partner deserve peace and happiness.

CHAPTER 10

LOVE HAS NO AGE

"Everyone is the age of their heart."

—Guatemalan proverb

When we think of the single lifestyle, we imagine the promiscuous but baffled 20-something-year-old characters of HBO's *Girls* or the fluctuating sexually confident or insecure mid-30s foursome of *Sex and the City*—women and men living in cities, following their dreams by day and going to clubs at night, either playing the field or desperately searching for life partners and mates. It may come as a shock to learn that today, *more than 45 percent of single people in the U.S. are over the age of 50*![1]

More people are getting divorced after the age of 50 than ever before.[2]

The baby boomers—the post–World War II generation, born between 1946 to 1964—have changed the fabric of society at every stage of their lives, in every decade they've lived through, and they're changing it again now, even as their hair is getting gray.

As the baby boomers age, we are witnessing a sea change in the way older people approach sexuality and aging. One reason for this is our desire to live longer—plus all the medical and scientific progress that has helped us remain healthy and vital. Another factor is that more of us reject the arbitrary mandate to retire at 65 from work we are passionate about. We want to stay young and productive as long as we're alive. We realize that we have a lifetime of wisdom that makes these last few decades of our time on earth even more valuable, not just to us but to those we love and the world at large. Those of us who are baby boomers aren't about to consign ourselves to golf, gardening, and soap operas for the last few decades of our lives. We still have life to live and lots of work to do.

Another important factor leading to change has been women's evolving self-perception. Before the beginning of the feminist movement, prior generations relegated older women to a dependent position—practically rendering them invisible. Today, this is no longer the case. Just think of all the vibrant, inspiring role models we see around us who are 60 or older: former IBM CEO Meg Whitman; present IBM CEO, Ginni Rometty; media mogul, philanthropist, and actress Oprah Winfrey; former presidential candidate and secretary of state Hillary Clinton; fashion icon Diane Von Furstenberg; Dr. Ruth Westheimer and newswoman Barbara Walters—both in their 80s; and actress and animal activist Betty White, who is 95! These women are all energetic, vital, and more productive than most men and women in their 30s. It's clear that women in the later decades have started to see themselves through a different prism. They are wiser and smarter, and want to maintain if not enhance their usefulness to society after their children are grown and have left the home. As women age, they find themselves free from many of the pressures society previously placed on them—pressure to be ornamental sexual objects, pressure to be selfless mothers, pressure to be subservient and accept the role of second-class citizens. They have a heightened awareness of their own needs, which builds confidence and makes them less likely to settle for second best or resign themselves to a life devoid of romance, sexuality, and intimacy.

So let's not look at being single as we age as a sad situation. It is just another phase, and the better prepared and more comfortable we are with ourselves, the more likely we are to enjoy this phase—and perhaps even make it the most significant time of our lives. This isn't to say that there isn't trauma associated with splitting up or losing a partner after many decades; it's just that now, we have more options. Baby boomer women and men are part of a brave new generation that continues to transform the way the world works.

BABY BOOMERS BY THE NUMBERS

- A 50-year-old female can expect to live 82.5 years; a male, 78.5 years.[3]
- Over 74.9 million baby boomers are 50+.[4]
- By the year 2030, baby boomers will be ages 66 to 84 and make up 20 percent of the total population.[5]
- Boomers work past retirement. Only 11 percent plan to stop working entirely. A survey by AARP reveals most boomers plan to work "until they drop."[6]
- 109 percent of all baby boomers are divorced.[7]
- December 31, 2029 is the day the last of the baby boomers will turn 65.[8]

Maggie started seeing me soon after she went into menopause in her early 50s. Smart, interesting, and powerful, she ran a major advertising agency employing hundreds of workers. She and her second husband, Sean, had been happily married for 20 years. One day, their life changed. Sean had a stroke, leaving him severely handicapped. For more than a decade, Maggie took care of Sean, their six children, and eight grandchildren, until the day when, loving family by his side, Sean died peacefully at home. While death never comes at the right time and Maggie struggled to accept her devastating loss, the great support of family and friends and the wonderfully fulfilling life she had built helped carry her through the grieving process.

"In retrospect, the last few years of Sean's life were even harder than his passing. I was at work all day long, then home at night putting all my energies into trying to make Sean feel better and keeping the family together. Intimacy through sex were things of the past," she explained. "I felt so bad for Sean, and I was so busy with my work, kids, and life in general, I never thought I was missing something.

"When Sean passed, my friends and family were constantly around and full of love and support, making sure I was busy and never alone. As the months passed, some of my support system thought it was time for me to get back into the dating world. I had absolutely no interest and told them I wasn't ready. To be honest, I never saw romance in my future. I thought myself lucky to have had such an amazing life with Sean, and was just grateful for that.

"One thing about life—it is full of surprises. About a year after Sean died, I went on a trip to the Bahamas with some friends. That's where I met Paul. He is a poet and an artist, a few years my junior. Paul was vacationing at the same resort, and one day by the pool we started talking. To my surprise, he lived in the same town I do. Within a few days we became fast friends, and before I went back home we exchanged phone numbers. He called while I was still at the airport getting my bags and invited me to an art exhibit. Of course I said yes, and since then—it's a year now—I've been spending all my free time with him. I knew from the moment we started talking by the pool that this man and I had chemistry. Turns out I was right. I can't tell you how strange it was the first time we made love. I couldn't imagine taking my clothes off in front of a strange man. We were both older, and I never saw an older body on a TV or movie screen, so I never thought old could be sexy. I felt scared and embarrassed. I wanted all the lights out, got into bed and covered myself to my nose; was so scared and embarrassed, I could barely believe I was going to do this. But he was so gentle and so caring that within a few minutes I relaxed and let myself go. He liked my body and strangely I found his sexy too. Things heated up between us with lightning speed. Turns out he is a fantastic lover. In fact, I doubt I've ever had sex like the sex we have together. We stay up all night and spend weekends in bed just having sex and playing. It's amazing this is happening to me at this age. And he is a magnificent companion and always interesting to be with and talk to. My friends and family all think he's great, and they are very happy for us both. We spend a lot of time together and just like teens, we always wind up making out or just having sex. It's the funniest and strangest thing all at once."

When Maggie came to see me around the time she and Paul were marking their six-month anniversary, I almost didn't recognize her. Maggie had lost 10 pounds, was wearing bright and sexy clothes, and had cut her hair and dyed it a beautiful shade of auburn. She was beaming and looked like a 30-year-old. Maggie, usually a very private person, couldn't stop talking about the excitement the new relationship and her new man were bringing her.

"My sex life is fantastic. I feel open and loved. Now I cannot believe that I had no interest in sex for so many years. I have no idea what the future holds for Paul and me, but strangely, I'm not worried about the future. I've never been happier and wouldn't trade this time of my life for anything in the world. I'm alive again. For the longest time, I thought feeling this way wasn't in the cards for our age group."

From my professional and personal experience, I can tell you Maggie's story is not so unique. Fairy tales like this do happen in real life, and it makes me so happy I want to share them with you. I wish this kind of awakening for all my single patients, regardless of their age. Sex certainly brings back the desire to live, flirt, be noticed, and notice life in its brightest colors. It takes away the daily drudgery too many of us put up with for far too long.

Like Maggie, Maria also found rejuvenating love again—at age 72.

"Mark is probably my last love," the silver-haired beauty told me. "Ironically, he and I dated briefly five decades ago, but he moved across the country for a job and we lost touch. We both married different people and had families. I had a great marriage for 35 years, but my husband passed away. A few years later—after I'd pretty much resigned myself to being alone forever—Mark and I reconnected on Facebook. Turns out he was divorced and free—and we were living in the same state! We started e-mailing, then talking on the phone, and soon we made a date to meet in person. When we first saw each other, it was a little shocking—we each noticed immediately how much the other had aged! But the most beautiful and unexpected thing happened. Within a few hours of talking and reminiscing, the time seemed to vanish from our faces. I always used to wonder how older people maintain passionate love, and now I know—they don't see each other as old. Mark and I just picked up where we had left off half a century earlier. Our relationship is everything I could have wished for. We do have sex, but at our age, we both need some pharmaceutical help. He takes testosterone and Viagra, and I take testosterone too for my sex drive and lubrication. But it is our intimacy and passion that make sex so great and life together so full. I am a lucky woman, and he is a lucky man! What a great fortune to get another chance!"

For those who are older and more experienced, and whose lives have lots of history, it is important to realize that sex can bring back long-forgotten feelings. Between the sex-charged teens and 20s to that commitment-filled time of life when raising a family places the needs of others before one's own, sex is often lost in translation. When people have found themselves devoid of really passionate, intimate sex for decades, it invariably is a wonderful, life-affirming experience when it returns.

Sometimes that sexual rejuvenation happens within the structure of a longtime marriage, when the kids leave and two people rekindle the spark that brought them together in the first place. But there are others who suffer through life without sex and intimacy in cold, loveless marriages, which often feels worse than being alone.

Jean, a 53-year-old nurse, has been starved for intimacy for too long. She raised four children over the course of a 30-year marriage, and her relationship with her husband, Todd, a cold and emotionally unavailable man, is nothing more than an arrangement. She freely admits that Todd's only redeeming quality is that he earns a lot of money and provides her with a luxurious lifestyle, holding her back from walking out. On the rare occasions that Todd is home, he spends his time watching TV, reading on his iPad, or texting.

"Quality time? What's that?" Jean asked me, her voice tinged with resentment. "The kids are gone and they rarely come to see us. Todd and I don't talk. He sits on the couch staring at some electronic gadget or goes to bed early. We've slept in different bedrooms for more than a decade now. I originally asked him to move out because of his snoring, since there was no sex anyway and we weren't emotionally close enough to even cuddle with each other. Once in a while he would come to my bedroom and we'd have half-hearted sex, but there was no real passion or intimacy there. Over time, neither one of us made an effort any more, so sex died out altogether. Now it's just a big, cold house with two people in it; we're roommates who don't even like each other. I see him like a piece of furniture. The kids feel the lack of warmth in our house. I'm sure they couldn't wait to grow up and move out. I certainly would if I could. Every one of them chose a college as far away from home as possible. When I want to see my kids, I go to their homes. Todd sometimes comes along, but we all know he isn't really interested in them or their lives. He is so closed off.

"It's not as if I haven't tried working on the marriage. Initially I did everything I knew to save it. I went to a therapist, hoping to figure out what I was doing wrong. After 10 years, the therapist told me if I wanted a loving husband, I was barking up the wrong tree with Todd. I pleaded with Todd to go to couples therapy, so he agreed and went a few times just so I would stop nagging him. He was totally dismissive of the process, saying there wasn't anything therapy could teach him. It took me years to accept the fact that he wasn't going to change and turn into a loving and open-hearted man.

"A few years ago, I went on a Caribbean getaway with a few of my girlfriends and I hooked up with another vacationer. In spite of all the possible downsides of the fling—like catching an STD or getting found out by Todd—I suddenly felt alive. After the fling, I was young again. Life was great again, and all the sadness and frustration of life with Todd were gone. I think at that point there was a shift in me, and suddenly I felt I was single again and no longer tied by the marriage vows to Todd.

"Last year, I started an affair closer to home with a doctor at our local hospital. It's still going strong, but here's the thing: While it's exciting and dangerous, it's not much more than sex. It's good sex but it's not intimate. It's not love; it just fills part of the hole my marriage has left in my life. For now, this is good enough, although a little too close for comfort, but I am still optimistic the right man will come along. When he does, then maybe I'll get the courage to leave this marriage and have what I've always dreamed of—both passionate sex and an intimate relationship. I still believe I'm owed a knight in shining armor in this lifetime."

For others, compromise within the marriage is the best option. My patient Melanie, 62, shared her story. "You know that middle-aged couple in the restaurant who sit through a three-course meal without saying a word to one another? That was me.

"When I married Jack, we were in our 30s. We were both successful professionals with great jobs, so we were able to build a really great life together. Neither one of us had the desire to have a family. We loved being alone, so we decided not to have children. From the first date on, the chemistry between us was great and we spent all our free time having sex. The initial five years of our marriage can be described as 'sex, sex, sex, and more sex.' But once that passion started to fade, it started to be clear that we actually had very little else in common. Our careers kept us busy and out of the house so much that we were able to avoid facing the fact that the only thing holding the marriage together had been sex. As we aged, sex started to lose its importance. I went into menopause and lost my libido; Jack went into male menopause and became a grouch. We both started to look for excuses not to be with one another. We really never learned to communicate in the earlier years of our relationship, so there were a lot of deadly silences whenever we did spend time together. Once sex was gone, there was no warmth or cuddling or anything that could be used to pass for intimacy between us.

"Initially that was very disturbing to me, and I thought the marriage was doomed and I would have to move on. But as I've grappled with this frustration for a long time, I eventually reached a compromise I can live with. With Jack, my life is peaceful and comfortable. We don't argue, and we still present ourselves as a couple to the outside world, which has become very important as we got older and our social life has risen to higher socioeconomic levels with VIPs and celebrities. I never thought I could live without sex and intimacy, but I found that it's quite possible. I think I'm living a double life where a part of me is alone and another part is a couple. Jack is a nice man; he treats me respectfully and kindly, and he does love me in his own way. Life with him is good, and I don't want to hurt him by seeking sex or passion outside the marriage. The compromise is good and I don't feel I compromised myself, since I have had a fulfilling and sex-filled life before Jack and even with Jack. I just think this is a good and sound way to allow age to settle in."

Melanie's compromise is the most commonly chosen option I have encountered in my decades of listening to men and women talk about their relationships and marriages as they age. There seems to be a point in a person's life when he or she makes the decision to stop looking, to stop hoping that something better is around the corner, and just accepts the status quo, calling it the reality of life. Whether the person is single or married doesn't matter. In our society, where being part of a couple is perceived as the norm, many couples stay together just for show, as an arrangement of convenience rather than as a passionate, loving, and connected twosome. If that works without compromising yourself and you are on the same page with your partner with common interests and like each other, it may be time to call it a good marriage.

A NEW PERSPECTIVE ON SEXUAL PARTNERS

Most people do what is expected of them, just like their parents, and their parents' parents, and everyone around them has always done. They marry, build families, and have children and raise them, regardless of whether those life choices are theirs consciously or just imposed by societal rules. Once that phase is over, they are free to express their sexuality in different ways. Faith is one such woman who has gone this route. Her life changed dramatically after her husband of 40 years died.

"I was such a traditional wife and mother," Faith, 67, explained. "I was expected to marry a good provider, and I did. I was expected to have and raise children, and I did. My life was not unlike that of my parents; it was very safe. Bill and I were always social and spent much of our married life mingling with other couples. We went out to dinner, on vacations, to church functions, even joined the local golf-and-racket club. We were always on the go. And yet, looking back on that life, there was something missing in me that I never took the time to explore or understand. I loved Bill, but I never found him sexually exciting. I was a virgin when we married, so I had no idea what sex or love was about. I read books and watched TV, secretly wondering what all the fuss was about sex. When Bill passed away, I felt lost. I rapidly found myself following the lifestyle of an elderly widow. I babysat the grandchildren, prepared holiday dinners, and went to the movies with other widows and divorced friends. That phase lasted a year.

"One morning, after having watched a passion-filled independent movie the night before, I made the decision to go back to school, to learn more about art. Art seemed to be the expression of passion, and passion was what I had been missing my entire life. That's where I met Rita. She was a 55-year-old attractive single brunette who had been successful in finance and wanted to pursue a more creative career. Her goal was to run an art gallery; she knew the business end but needed some art courses. We were both changing direction at this point in our lives, and we hit it off right away. We started going for coffee after class, then out to dinner almost every night, and we became great friends, sharing everything about ourselves with each other. One evening, we were studying for an exam at her apartment. She suddenly put her hands on my shoulders and turned me towards her. She gently caressed my face and started kissing me. At first, I was shocked. I never thought of myself as a lesbian, but in that moment, I realized I was more sexually attracted to this woman than I had ever been to my husband for 40 years. The passion was overwhelming, and sex was amazing! We have been inseparable since that evening. We now live together, and I finally understand what I missed for all the years I was married to Bill. My relationship with Rita encompasses everything. It is friendship, love, sex, intimacy; it's what I envisioned a true relationship would be."

SEXUAL FLUIDITY

A few years ago, a patient came to see me and told me a story unlike anything I'd heard before. Diane was in her mid-40s and described herself as very sexual. She said sex had always been of utmost importance to her.

As a young woman, Diane had gone to an all-female college and, while not identifying herself as gay, had fallen in love with a girl down the hall in her dorm. A brief but torrid love affair with the woman made her assume she was a lesbian, and she immediately told her parents. While initially a bit disappointed—Diane was the first in their mostly conservative family to profess same-sex interest—they loved their daughter and were nonetheless supportive. They even invited Diane's college girlfriend over for Thanksgiving dinner. Throughout her college years, Diane enjoyed a few more short affairs with women.

By the time she graduated college, Diane told me, the blush of excitement over sex with women had faded, and to her surprise, she found herself attracted to Roland, a man in her graduate school program. They fell in love, and, by the time they married, Diane chalked her history of sexual relations with women up to college experimentation. On her wedding night, she was 100 percent sure she was heterosexual.

Diane had two children with her husband and was happy for at least a decade with both her marriage and their sex life. But as time passed, she started to feel that her relationship with her husband was becoming stale. While her sex drive was still extremely strong, she no longer found her husband attractive.

To her shock, she realized she was obsessively lusting after her closest female friend. This was confusing, to say the least, especially since she knew her girlfriend was straight. She didn't want to lose the friendship, and spent sleepless nights wondering if her girlfriend could possibly feel the same way, or if she'd be appalled or angry if Diane spoke up about her feelings. As she was trying to figure out what to do with her newfound passion, she also started to doubt the need for her marriage to continue.

Diane and her husband were close friends and had always communicated well during their marriage, and Roland figured out that something was off. When Diane admitted she was having fantasies about her girlfriend, he promptly took them both to a marriage and family therapist. The therapist was very helpful, giving the couple new insight into the sexuality of women.

The therapist told the couple that women in general had a much more fluid perspective on sexuality than men. According to the therapist—and this is backed up by current biological and psychological research on sexuality—women don't need to identify themselves as straight, lesbian, or bisexual. Many women just move between loving a man or a woman with ease. Women are more likely to connect deep feelings of love to a person, not a specific gender.

IS SEXUAL FLUIDITY FOR REAL?

Lisa Diamond, a University of Utah psychology professor, has studied the phenomenon extensively for her book, *Sexual Fluidity: Understanding Women's Love and Desire.*

She sees sexual fluidity as having three defining characteristics:

- Nonexclusivity in attractions: can find either gender sexually attractive
- Changes in attractions: can suddenly find a man or woman sexually attractive after having been in a long-term relationship with the other
- Attraction to a person, not the gender

In a 2008 study, Diamond reported on 70 lesbian, bisexual, and "unlabeled" women over the course of 10 years. During that decade:

- Two-thirds changed their initial sexual identity labels.
- One-third changed labels at least twice.
- Overall the most commonly adopted sexual identity was "unlabeled."

According to data compiled by the Williams Institute,[9] an independent UCLA think tank focusing on gender studies and public policy, far more female survey subjects reported incidents of same-sex attraction and sexual behaviors during their lifetime than did those who identified themselves as lesbian, gay, or bisexual. An estimated 19 million Americans (8.2 percent) reported that they have engaged in same-sex sexual behavior, and nearly 25.6 million Americans (11 percent) acknowledged at least some same-sex sexual attraction.

Computational neuroscientists Ogi Ogas and Sai Gaddam, authors of the fascinating book *A Billion Wicked Thoughts: What the Internet Tells Us About Sexual Relationships*, have studied the brain and how it reacts to sexual arousal, and related those studies to the online porn and erotica habits of millions of men and women. They discovered that as far as brain functions went, straight, gay, and bisexual men were far more likely to choose one sexual preference than women regarding what turned them on. Across the board, men were very simple in terms of their arousal cues. Visuals of women's breasts, sexual organs, men and women having intercourse, women having intercourse or kissing other women, or the suggestion of the possibility of intercourse caused arousal in the majority of healthy men. Women, on the other hand, were far more complex and needed a mix of different cues in order to become aroused. While men across the spectrum used pornography extensively as a source of arousal, only between 8 to 20 percent of women even found porn interesting in terms of their sexual response. [10]

Diane was unique among the many women I've met—not because she allowed herself to be sexually fluid, but because she was so *clear* about it. She accepted who she was and lived her life without self-judgment or fear of repercussions or disapproval from her peer group. She didn't go back to love affairs with women but always had close and very loving, though asexual, relationships with the women in her life. But her story took another interesting twist. As she aged, she developed sexual feelings for another man and began an affair, one that was so intense that it threatened to upend her marriage to Roland, who by this time had become an old roommate. The players in this drama came up with an unexpected compromise: Diane's lover moved in with Diane and her husband, raising the kids in their now extended, albeit unconventional, family. Both men were at peace with the arrangement, and my patient described a very gratifying, sex-filled life with the two men she loved dearly.

Diane's story may sound extreme to you, but continuing research into sexual fluidity and the variations in human sexual response indicates that elements of it may not be that uncommon after all.[11]

Maybe the lesson here is that love and lust are about individual people, not about gender-specific labels—and as long as the parties involved share similar interests and accept each other, the situation can turn out to be a good thing.

THE STORY OF SEX...ISN'T JUST ABOUT SEX

As we've traveled through the life cycles of sexuality through patient stories, one thread ties together the wide variety of experiences from people of different backgrounds, races, and ages: Sexuality is influential at all ages but is an ever-changing dynamic, varying in importance and definition at different times throughout the journey of life. Sex can mean lust, a desire to just have fun, or the physical expression of both passion and deep caring. Sex can lie dormant for decades while other priorities loom larger, but even as sex hormones leave us during the aging process, it still remains a significant force in our lives, as a vehicle both for pure pleasure and for expressing our feelings of love and intimacy toward another human being.

During our hormone-charged youth and our reproductive years, sex is vital, when we are in love or when our desire for sex is reciprocated. Life without sex—when we feel unloved and abandoned and have no other way of connecting to another human—can feel tragic and empty. But despite what R- and X-rated movies, internet porn, and popular romance novels would have us believe, life without sex is perfectly fine too, as long as we are happy and feel emotionally fulfilled in other areas of our lives. Sex does not remain the same for anyone from the time he or she is an adolescent to old age—every person will weather multiple changes in his or her sexuality. At the end of the day, it is all about us as individuals and how we choose to live our lives. Sex may be a central part of being human, but it is not just about the body, about reproduction, or even about love. It must fit into the bigger picture of our personal choices and how we find a deeper emotional and spiritual satisfaction in life. Your family, your friends, and the media may try to convince you that you are somehow "doing it wrong," but living by committee or following someone else's life script never, ever leads to happiness.

It's your life—and your sex—so make it work for you.

EPILOGUE

The 1973 Ingmar Bergman movie *Scenes from a Marriage* tells the story of the disintegration of the marriage between Marianne, a lawyer, and Johan, a professor, over the course of more than a decade. Described by *Boxoffice* magazine as "painfully intimate, almost pornographically personal, Ingmar Bergman's masterful *Scenes from a Marriage* remains, more than three decades after its making, the best film ever made about relationships."

Initially a TV series, *Scenes from a Marriage* became notorious worldwide. Its impact was overwhelming. The divorce rate in Sweden rose significantly during the decade that followed its launch. Many other movies and TV series that followed were modeled on Ingmar Bergman's work of art and its raw honesty.

When I saw the movie, its effect was transformative. I understood that communication made a marriage work, that sex is a highly significant ingredient in a successful marriage. I also caught a glimpse of the amount of deception and manipulation involved in marriage and some insight into how personal growth determines outcome. I thought *Scenes from a Marriage* forced people to accept the truth about the underbelly of relationships, and helped set us free to live on our own terms moving toward our own personal truth in life and in relationships.

I found the impact of this movie long lasting even a decade later as a young woman, a doctor running a major trauma center in New York with a small baby and a husband. The movie took me out of my life and opened my eyes to a much more complex reality.

The movie helped me open the door to my personal freedom. Although my life is complex and full of contradictions and flaws, overall, it's a continuum of enlightening and wonderfully empowering experiences. It is a wonderful ride that I wish to share with you as a way of showing you we're all the same—in turmoil or at peace, we are always individuals creating our own lives. I hope my story brings you solace and kindness.

I was raised in Bucharest, Romania, during the era of Communism, by good parents. They wanted to prepare me for life by giving me a solid and extensive education and supporting me unconditionally. They gave me what we are all looking for: validation for all my cockamamie ideas and the tools to succeed. Amy Chua and Jed Rubenfeld's book *The Triple Package: How Three Unlikely Traits Explain the Rise and Fall of Cultural Groups in America* tells us about the trifecta that makes certain people and ethnic groups successful: a sense of superiority, insecurity, and persistence. My parents encouraged those traits in me since childhood. They taught me self-confidence, care for others and, above all, honesty and courage to face my personal truth in everything I did.

They raised me to be strong and fearless even though they launched me into a highly discriminatory man's world. I never heard about discrimination, racism, or women's liberation in my parents' home. To my parents, everyone was the same and the only goal was to help others and serve the greater good. The one pervasive message my father gave me was to be independent both financially and emotionally. He encouraged me to focus on my studies above everything else. Of course, I fell in love at 15 with a boy I went to high school with. That didn't please my dad, and he forbade me from seeing the boy. In Eastern Europe in the 1960s, parents were strict and children obeyed. While I was trying to figure out how to continue seeing my boyfriend without my parent's knowledge, my family moved to Italy making the entire situation moot.

In Rome, I went to an American high school, learned English and put my romantic dreams on the back burner. It was difficult, because, all around me, hormone-driven teens cared about only love, romance, and sex and I certainly was no different. Before I graduated high school and headed for New York, I did, however, meet a nice Italian boy willing to teach me the ways of puppy love Italian-style.

That was great for a few months yet before I could get immersed in the Italian experience, life took me across the ocean to New York and a new life. I didn't understand the American culture, but reading romance novels and watching movies filled in the blanks and fueled my teen romance fantasies.

I graduated college in New York and went on to medical school. Although medical education was of primary importance to me, I willingly followed the lead of friends and media. I started going out, and quickly my focus shifted to the company of boys.

My parents were strict and very afraid of my budding sexuality, and many a time my father would tell me to pay attention to my schoolwork rather than go out—because, as he said, "once you have sex, the guy will lose respect for you and you will never reach your goal to be a doctor." I wanted to be a doctor since I was five, and nothing was going to stop that, so I listened to his advice…as much as I could.

My Americanization started in college. I did well in school, and I also enjoyed my extracurricular activities. I started dating and had a blast. My father was nonplussed and set impossible curfews. I had to be home to the Upper East Side apartment I shared with my parents by 10 p.m.—an almost unattainable goal I was able to keep with few exceptions, when my mom and dad were waiting for me at the door, ready to ground me for life. Surprisingly, I survived and so did they. In time, they accepted my Americanization and loosened the reins.

By my third year in college, I had a steady boyfriend and even started having sex. There was no fear of STDs in those days, and the world was a simple place. The guys I dated wanted to marry me, and I had no idea how to say no. In fact, I doubt I had any idea about what relationships were. Just like everyone else my age, I thought good sex (whatever that meant) was equal to a good relationship.

While my main focus stayed on school and then on my work, I said yes more than once to the proposals, and found myself engaged and married without ever giving a thought to why I was doing it or what the long-term consequences would be. In fact, I never thought about what my relationships would look like 20 years down the line.

Fortunately, the men I sequentially married have been good guys, and, also fortunately, I have two wonderful girls, who are my best friends today.

My work in medicine and being a mother kept me so busy I focused more on those things than on my relationships with men.

Although sex has always been important to me, it didn't define who I was or whether I would stay with a man. Each time I got divorced, it had nothing to do with sex. It was more about my outgrowing the relationship and listening to my personal truth, which told me I would be better off moving on than staying and making everyone miserable.

As my career grew and my patients shared their personal lives with me, I realized that while sexuality is highly important and we need it to have children and fun, unless it is tied into a good relationship that keeps us connected with common interests and mutual support and acceptance, it really is just window dressing. Disconnected from emotions it is but a series of positions in Kama Sutra pictures or porn videos.

As a woman, a practicing physician, mother and grandmother I see life as all about love, and sex as one of the many manifestations of love.

Love defines us and sex serves a very important role in our expression of love, lust and passion at various stages and phases of our life.

I hope this book helps you gain a better understanding of the connection between love, sex, intimacy and fun in your own life.

Thank you.

RECOMMENDED READING

Why Men Fake It: The Totally Unexpected Truth about Men and Sex, by Abraham Morgentaler, MD.

Testosterone for Life: Recharge Your Vitality, Sex Drive, Muscle Mass, and Overall Health, by Abraham Morgentaler, MD.

The Triple Package: How Three Unlikely Traits Explain the Rise and Fall of Cultural Groups in America, by Amy Chua and Jed Rubenfeld.

How We Do It: The Evolution and Future of Human Reproduction, by Robert Martin.

Sexual Behavior in the Human Male, by Alfred Kinsey.

Human Sexual Inadequacy, by William Masters and Virginia Johnson.

A Billion Wicked Thoughts: What the Internet Tells Us about Sexual Relationships, by Ogi Ogas and Sai Gaddam.

The Trouble with Testosterone: And Other Essays on the Biology of the Human Predicament, by Robert M. Sapolsky.

ENDNOTES

CHAPTER 1

1   Mona Chalabi, "How Many People Haven't Had Sex in the past Month?" *The Guardian*, January 24, 2014, http://www.theguardian.com/news/reality-check/2014/jan/24/how-many-people-havent-had-sex.

2   Sarah Jio, "Sex by the Numbers," *Woman's Day*, March 3, 2015, http://www.womansday.com/sex-relationships/sex-tips/sex-by-the-numbers-103274.

3   Jesse Bering, "Are There Asexuals among Us? On the Possibility of a 'Fourth' Sexual Orientation," *Scientific American Blog Network*, October 29, 2009, http://blogs.scientificamerican.com/bering-in-mind/2009/10/29/are-there-asexuals-among-us-on-the-possibility-of-a-fourth-sexual-orientation/.

CHAPTER 2

1   Harm Kuipers, "Anabolic Steroids: Side Effects," *Encyclopedia of Sports Medicine and Science*, March 7, 1998, http://www.sportsci.org/encyc/anabstereff/anabstereff.html.

G. Glazer, "Atherogenic Effects of Anabolic Steroids on Serum Lipid Levels. A Literature Review," *Archives of Internal Medicine*,

October 1991, PMID: 1929679, http://www.ncbi.nlm.nih.gov/ pubmed/1929679.

2   Jay Hoffman and Nicholas Ratamess, "Medical Issues Associated with Anabolic Steroid Use: Are They Exaggerated?" *Journal of Sports Science and Medicine* 5, no. 2 (2006): 182–193, PMCID: PMC3827559, https://www.ncbi.nlm.nih.gov/pmc/articles/ PMC3827559/.

CHAPTER 3

1   Tamar Lewin, "Are These Parties for Real?" *New York Times*, Fashion & Style, June 30, 2005, http://www.nytimes. com/2005/06/30/fashion/thursdaystyles/are-these-parties-for-real.html.

2   http://www.statejournal.com/story/17334114/ report-evidence-shows-abstinence-programs-don't-work Laura Stepp, "Study Casts Doubt on Abstinence-Only Programs," *The Washington Post*, April 14, 2007, http://www. washingtonpost.com/wp-dyn/content/article/2007/04/13/ AR2007041301003.html.

3   CDC

4   WHO bulletin "Human papillomavirus and HPV vaccines: a review," FT Cutts a, S Franceschi b, S Goldie c, et.al

5   Jonathan Benson, "Young Woman's Ovaries Destroyed by Gardasil: Merck 'Forgot to Research' Effects of Vaccine on Female Reproduction," *NaturalNews*, August 6, 2013, http://www.natu-ralnews.com/041512_gardasil_ovary_destruction_hpv_vaccine; http://healthimpactnews.com/2013/studyhpv-vaccine-linked-to-premature-menopause-in-young-girls/, and http://www.

trueactivist.com/its-official-139-girls-have-died-from-hpv-vacci-nations/.

6   "Med Alerts" *National Vaccine Information Center*, VAERS, May 21, 2017, http://www.nvic.org/Vaccines-and-Diseases/hpv.aspx.

7   "Judicial Watch Reports 371 Serious Adverse Events From Gardasil," *FDAnews Drug Daily Bulletin*, June 1, 2007, fdanews.com/articles/94086-judicial-watch-reports-371-serious-adverse-events-from-gardasil.

8   Gregory Poland, "Vaccines against Lyme Disease: What Happened and What Lessons Can We Learn?" Clinical Infectious Diseases 52, no. 3.1 (2011): s253–s258, https://doi.org/10.1093/cid/ciq116.

9   *Judicial Watch*, "Govt. Still Pushing HPV Vaccine on Kids a Decade after JW Exposed Deadly Side Effects," March 9 ,2017, https://www.judicialwatch.org/blog/2017/03/govt-still-pushing-hpv-vaccine-kids-decade-jw-exposed-deadly-side-effects/.

10 HIV Update 2017, published date April 28 2017, https://aidsetc.org/resource/hiv-update-2017.

11 *Centers for Disease Control and Prevention*, "Youth Risk Behavior Surveillance—United States, 2011," *MMWR* 61, no. 4 (2012): 1–162, https://www.cdc.gov/mmwr/preview/mmwrhtml/ss6104a1.htm.

12 *Centers for Disease Control and Prevention*, "Diagnoses of HIV Infection and AIDS in the United States and Dependent Areas," *HIV Surveillance Report* 21, (2009), https://www.cdc.gov/hiv/pdf/library/reports/surveillance/cdc-hiv-surveillance-report-2009-vol-21.pdf.

13 H. Weinstock, S. Berman, and W. Cates, Jr., "Sexually Transmitted Diseases Among American Youth: Incidence and Prevalence Estimates, 2000," *Perspectives on Sexual and Reproductive Health* 36, no. 1 (2004): 6–10, doi: 10.1363/psrh.36.6.04, https://www.ncbi.nlm.nih.gov/pubmed/14982671.

CHAPTER 4

1   J. Mascaro, P. Hackett, and J. Rilling, "Testicular Volume Is Inversely Correlated with Nurturing-Related Brain Activity in Human Fathers," *Proceedings of the National Academy of Science of the United States of America* 110. no. 39 (2013): 15748-17575, doi:10.1073/pnas.1305579110, https://www.ncbi.nlm.nih.gov/pubmed/24019499.

2   William Cromie, "Marriage Lowers Testosterone," *Harvard Gazette*, August 22, 2002, https://news.harvard.edu/gazette/story/2002/08/marriage-lowers-testosterone/.

3   L. Gettler et al., "Fatherhood, Childcare, and Testosterone: Study Authors Discuss the Details," *Scientific American*, October 5, 2011, https://blogs.scientificamerican.com/guest-blog/fatherhood-childcare-and-testosterone-study-authors-discuss-the-details/.

4   Bret Schulte, "How Common are Cheating Spouses," *US News*, March 27,2008, https://www.usnews.com/news/national/articles/2008/03/27/how-common-are-cheating-spouses.

5   J. Peterson and J. Hyde, "Gender Differences in Sexual Attitudes and Behaviors: A Review of Meta-Analytic Resuts and Large Datasets," *Journal of Sex Research* 48, no. 2–3 (2011): 149-165,

doi: 10.1080/00224499.2011.551851, https://www.ncbi.nlm.nih.
gov/pubmed/21409712.

6   PubMed.gov, *The Journal of Sexual Medicine*, October 3, 2017,
    epub, https://www.ncbi.nlm.nih.gov/pubmed/28986148.

7   Ji Hyun Lee, "Modern Lessons From Arranged Marriages,"
    The New York Times, January 18, 2013, http://www.nytimes.
    com/2013/01/20/fashion/weddings/parental-involvement-
    can-help-in-choosing-marriage-partners-experts-say.
    html?pagewanted=all&_r=0.

8   Dan Hurley, "Divorce Rate: It's Not as High as You Think,"
    The New York Times, April 19, 2005, http://www.nytimes.
    com/2005/04/19/health/19divo.html?_r=0.

9   "Divorce Rate Dropping—Unless You're a
    Baby Boomer," *American News Report*, Decem-
    ber 11, 2013, http://americannewsreport.com/
    divorce-rate-dropping-unless-youre-a-baby-boomer-8820318.

10 en.wikipedia.org/wiki/Birth_control.

11 M. Littleton, "The Truth About 'The Pill' and your Sex Drive,"
    WebMD, 2015 https://www.webmd.com/sex/birth-control/
    features/the-pill-and-desire.

12 Kelli Hall et al., "Studying the Use of Oral Contraception: A
    Review of Measurement Approaches," *Journal of Women's Health*
    19. no. 10 (2010): 2203–2210, doi: 10.1089/jwh.2010.1963,
    https://www.ncbi.nlm.nih.gov/pmc/articles/PMC2990281/.

13 "Why Is Potentially Lethal Contraceptive Nuvaring Still on the
    Market?" *Vanity Fair*, December 9, 2013, https://www.vanityfair.
    com/news/2013/12/nuvaring-birth-control-investigation.

CHAPTER 5

1   Janell Fetterolf, "In Many Countries, at Least Four-in-Ten in the Labor Force are Women," PEW RESEARCH CENTER, March 2017, http://www.pewresearch.org/fact-tank/2017/03/07/in-many-countries-at-least-four-in-ten-in-the-labor-force-are-women/.

2   Marianne Bertrand, Emir Kamenica, and Jessica Pan, "Gender Identity and Relative Income within Households," *The Quarterly Journal of Economics* (2015): 571–614, doi: 10.1093/qje/qjv001, http://faculty.chicagobooth.edu/emir.kamenica/documents/identity.pdf.

3   M. Douglas, "Part 1: The Past, Present, and Future Wedding Industry," *Huffpost*, February 23, 2017, huffingtonpost.com/matt-douglas/part-1-the-past-present-f_b_9294420.html.

4   L. Ali, "The Curious Lives of Surrogates," *Newsweek*, March 29, 2008 http://www.newsweek.com/curious-lives-surrogates-84469.

5   "Relationships in America," topcounselingschools.org, www.topcounselingschools.org/relationships-in-america.

6   www.ncbi.nlm.nih.gov/pubmed/8516669.

7   www.livescience.com/1135-wild-sex-monogamy-rare.html.

8   Michael Balter, "Monogamy May Have Evolved to Prevent Infanticide," *Science*, July 29, 2013, http://news.sciencemag.org/brain-behavior/2013/07/monogamy-may-have-evolved-prevent-infanticide.

9   www.reuters.com/article/us-science-monogamy/for-males-monogamy-can-have-evolutionary-benefits-idUSBRE96S0XE20130729.

10 Carl Zimmer, "Monogamy and Human Evolution," *The New York Times*, August 2, 2013, http://www.nytimes.

com/2013/08/02/science/monogamys-boost-to-human-evolu-tion.html?_r=0.

11 Brian Switek, "Cheating and Divorce among Gibbons," Entertaining Research, November 13, 2007, http://mogadalai.wordpress.com/2007/11/13/cheating-and-divorce-among-gibbons/.

12 Christopher Ryan, "Monogamy Unnatural for Our Sexy Species," CNN, July 29, 2010, http://www.cnn.com/2010/OPINION/07/27/ryan.promiscuity.normal/index.html.

13 Clare Tanton et al., "Patterns and Trends in Sources of Information about Sex among Young People in Britain: Evidence from Three National Surveys on Sexual Attitudes and Lifestyles," *BMJ* 5, no. 3 (2015), doi: 10.1136/bmjopen-2015-007834, http://dx.doi.org/10.1136/bmjopen-2015-007834.

CHAPTER 6

1 A. Cherlin, "Demographic Trends in the United States: A Review of Research in the 2000s," *J Marriage Fam*, 2010 June; 72(3):403-419.

2 E. Lisitsa, "The Four Horsemen: Criticism, Contempt, Defensiveness, and Stonewall", The Gottman Relation-ship Blog, April 24, 2013, https://www.gottman.com/blog/the-four-horsemen-recognizing-criticism-contempt-defensive-ness-and-stonewalling/.

3 John Gottman, "The Gottman Institute," www.gottman.com. E. Lisitsa, "The Research: Predicting Divorce from Oral Historview Interview," The Gottman

Institute, https://www.gottman.com/blog/
the-research-predicting-divorce-from-an-oral-history-interview/.

4   Cory Silverberg, "Myths about Masturbation," *LiveAbout*, February 15, 2017, http://sexuality.about.com/od/masturbation/tp/
masturbationmyt.htm.

5   Harriet Hogarth and Roger Ingram, "Masturbation among Young Women and Associations with Sexual Health: An Exploratory Study," *The Journal of Sex Research* 46, no. 6 (2009): 558–567, http://www.tandfonline.com/doi/
full/10.1080/00224490902878993.

CHAPTER 7

1   "Low Sperm Count," *Mayo Clinic*, July 15, 2015, www.mayo-clinic.org/diseases-conditions/low-sperm-count/basics/causes/
con-20033441.

2   Lori Gottlieb, "Does a More Equal Marriage Mean Less Sex?" *The New York Times*, February 6, 2014, http://www.nytimes.
com/2014/02/09/magazine/does-a-more-equal-marriage-mean-less-sex.html.

3   Catherine Rampell, "Woman as Family Breadwinner on the Rise Study Says," *The New York Times*, May 29, 2013, http://www.
nytimes.com/2013/05/30/business/economy/women-as-family-breadwinner-on-the-rise-study-says.html.

4   Sabino Kornrich, Julie Brines, and Katrina Leupp, "Egalitarianism, Housework, and Sexual Frequency in Marriage," *American Sociological Review* 78, no. 1 (2012): 26–50, doi: 10.1177/0003122412472340, http://www.asanet.org/journals/
ASR/Feb13ASRFeature.pdf.

CHAPTER 8

1   Molly Edmonds, "Empty Nest Syndrome Overview," *HowStuff-Works*, February 18, 2009, http://health.howstuffworks.com/wellness/aging/empty-nest/empty-nest-syndrome2.htm.

2   "More Baby Boomer Marriages Going Bust," *American Academy of Matrimonial Lawyers*, August 2, 2016, http://aaml.org/about-the-academy/press/press-releases/more-baby-boomer-marriages-going-bust.

3   Susan Brown and I-Fen Lin, "The Gray Divorce Revolution: Rising Divorce Among Middle-Aged and Older Adults, 1990–2010," *Journals of Gerontology: Series B* 67, no. 6 (2012): 731–741, https://doi.org/10.1093/geronb/gbs089.

4   Ibid.

5   Elizabeth Bernstein, "The Loneliness of the Empty Nest," *The Wall Street Journal*, July 1, 2013, https://www.wsj.com/articles/SB10001424127887324436104578579372436143196.

CHAPTER 9

1   *Reviews in Urology*, "Testerosterone Replacement in Men with Andropause: An Overview," Michael K. Brawner, MD, ncbi.nlm.nih.gov/pmc/articles/PMC1472881/.

2   A. Morgentaler, M. Zitzmann, A. Traish, "Fundamental Concepts Regarding Testosterone Deficiency and Treatment: International Expert Consensus Resolutions," Mayo Clinic, July 2016, Vol. 91, Issue 7, Pg. 881-896.

3   C. Huggins and CV Hodges, "Studies On Prostatic Cancer: I. The Effect of Castration, of Estrogen and of Androgen Injection

On Serum Phosphatases in Metastatic Carcinoma of the Prostate." 1941. J Urol. 2002; 168:9–12.

4   A. Morgentaler, "Testostorone for Life: Recharge Your Vitality, Sex Drive, Muscle Mass, and Overall Health," Mcgraw-Hill Education, 1st Edition, November 17, 2008.

5   Luigi Ferrucci, Francesco Giallauria, and Jack Guralnik, "Epidemiology of Aging," Radiology Clinics of North America 46, no. 4 (2008): 643–652, doi: 10.1016/j.rcl.2008.07.005, https://pdfs.semanticscholar.org/0732/f7d30b4137d959fe5b-3d07134466b3d053c2.pdf.

6   T. Jeffrey, "First Time in Human History: People 65 and Older Will Outnumber Children Under 5," CNSnews.com, March 31,2016, https://www.cnsnews.com/news/article/terence-p-jeffrey/first-time-human-history-global-population-over-65-poised-pass.

7   "2009 National Survey of 5,045 Older Adults," *Journal of Sexual Medicine* 7, No. 5 (2010): 315–329.

8   Rabih Hijazi and Glenn Cunningham, "Andropause: Is Androgen Replacement Therapy Indicated for the Aging Male?" Annals of Rev Medicine 56 (2005): 117–137, http://www.annualreviews.org/doi/abs/10.1146/annurev.med.56.082103.104518.

CHAPTER 10

1   US Bureau of Labor Statistics (2014).

2   S. Roberts, "Divorce After 59 Grows More Common," *The New York Times*, Weddings, September 20, 2013.

3   The National Center for Health Statistics, 2010.
     S. Murphy, J. Xu, M.D., and K. Kochanek, "Deaths: Final Data

for 2015," National Vital Statistics for 2015, Vol. 66, Number 6, November 27, 2017.

4   Richard Fry, "Millenials Overtake Baby Boomers as America's. Largest Generation," *Pew Research Center*, Fact Tank, April 25, 2016, http://www.pewresearch.org/fact-tank/2016/04/25/millennials-overtake-baby-boomers/.

5   "Demographic Profile America's Older Boomers," *Metropolitan Life Insurance*, 2013, https://www.metlife.com/assets/cao/mmi/publications/Profiles/mmi-older-boomer-demographic-profile.pdf.

6   Jeff Love, "Approaching 65: A Survey of Baby Boomers Turning 65 Years Old," *AARP Research*, December 2010, https://www.aarp.org/research/topics/life/info-2014/approaching-65.html.

7   Renee Stepler, "Led by Baby Boomers, Divorce Rates Climb for America's 50+ Population," *Pew Research Center*, Fact Tank, March 9, 2017, http://www.pewresearch.org/fact-tank/2017/03/09/led-by-baby-boomers-divorce-rates-climb-for-americas-50-population/.

8   D'Vera Cohn and Paul Taylor, "Baby Boomers Approach 65—Glumly," *Pew Research Center*, Social & Demographic Trends, December 20, 2010, http://www.pewsocialtrends.org/2010/12/20/baby-boomers-approach-65-glumly/.

9   Gary Gates, "How Many People are Lesbian, Gay, Bisexual and Transgender," *The Williams Institute*, April 2011, https://williamsinstitute.law.ucla.edu/wp-content/uploads/Gates-How-Many-People-LGBT-Apr-2011.pdf.

10 Ogi Ogas and Sai Gaddam, *A Billion Wicked Thoughts: What the Internet Tells Us about Sexual Relationships* (Plume, 2011). http://www.billionwickedthoughts.com/science.html.

11   M. Nichols, "Lesbian sexuality/female sexuality: Rethinking 'lesbian bed death.'" Sexual and Relationship Therapy, Vol. 19, No. 4, November 2004, 363-371.

ABOUT THE AUTHOR

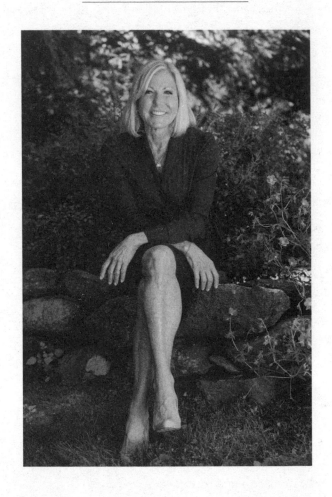

Erika Schwartz, MD, is an internationally acclaimed healthcare pioneer and key opinion leader in the field of prevention, hormones, and concierge and patient-centric medicine. A consummate clinician and patient advocate, Dr. Schwartz has cared for more than fifty thousand patients over forty years and is a highly sought after public speaker. Dr. Erika's groundbreaking book exposing the truth about our flawed health care system and empowering patients to take control over their own healthcare, *Don't Let Your Doctor Kill You* was published in November 2015 and *The New Hormone Solution* was published in May 2017.

Combining a Renaissance European upbringing, American education, passion for the patient, kindness, and common sense, Dr. Erika is the founder of Evolved Science, a concierge medical practice in New York City focused on exceptional and respectful patient services. Dr. Schwartz received her undergraduate degree with honors from New York University and her MD from SUNY-Downstate College of Medicine, Cum Laude. She is a member of Alpha Omega Alpha honor society and past president of the Board of Managers at SUNY-Downstate College of Medicine.

Dr. Erika is world renowned for her expertise and leadership in the conventional use of bioidentical hormones for women and men; supplements; patient advocacy; integration of diet, exercise, lifestyle; stress and relationship management and spiritual growth in all patient care. She is a firm believer that the doctor's role is to serve the patient. She believes public health and individualized care cannot be used interchangeably to improve our healthcare system and treat patients correctly.

Other Books
by ERIKA SCHWARTZ

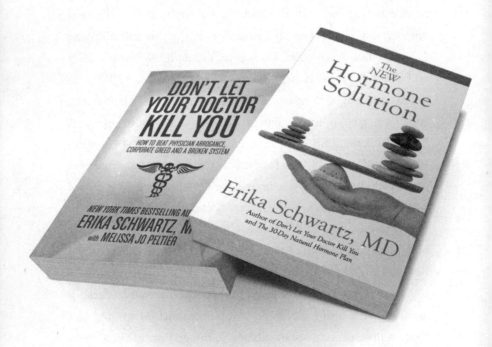

Don't Let Your Doctor Kill You
ISBN: 9781682613078
Price: USD $15.00 / CAD $20.00

The New Hormone Solution
ISBN: 9781682613306
Price: USD $16.00 / CAD $22.00

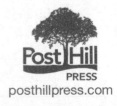